MW00449240

DIARY
OF A
CAREGIVER

DIARY
OF A
CAREGIVER

The Dementia Journey

REX T. YOUNG

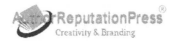
AuthorReputationPress®
Creativity & Branding

Copyright © 2021 by Rex T. Young

All rights reserved. No part of this publication may be reproduced, distributed, or transmitted in any form or by any means, including photocopying, recording, or other electronic or mechanical methods, without the prior written permission of the copyright owner and the publisher, except in the case of brief quotations embodied in critical reviews and certain other noncommercial uses permitted by copyright law. For permission requests, write to the publisher, addressed "Attention: Permissions Coordinator," at the address below.

Author Reputation Press LLC
45 Dan Road Suite 5
Canton MA 02021
www.authorreputationpress.com
Hotline: 1(800) 220-7660
Fax: 1(855) 752-6001

Ordering Information:
Quantity sales. Special discounts are available on quantity purchases by corporations, associations, and others. For details, contact the publisher at the address above.

Printed in the United States of America.

ISBN-13:	Softcover	978-1-64961-243-4
	eBook	978-1-64961-244-1

Library of Congress Control Number: 2021903184

CONTENTS

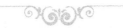

PREFACE

My wife has dementia with Alzheimer's symptoms. She was officially diagnosed in 2009 but looking back in time, there were signs in 2005 that I did not or chose not to recognize. As time passed the disease has worsened. As a caregiver, life has become more and more demanding. It is truly a 24 hour day and 7 day a week responsibility. If you have ever been involved in caregiving, you may recognized or be able to relate to some of the experiences that I have related. Some experiences are humorous at the time, some are humorous after the fact, and some can find no humor at all. For a new caregiver, this may be of no assistance at all, but it may alert you to what to expect.

I have not attempted to organize this diary in any particular order. My experiences and observations have been recorded as they occurred or came to light. It may appear rather chaotic but caregiving can certainly be that way.

I need some kind of project where I can keep my mind active and ponder what comes next. There are times when I am in the middle of a trying day or a trying time during a day when I can let my mind wander and try to compose, in my mind, what I would like to record of those experiences. I often refer to it as my sanity project.

We have been married since June 1958. Since our marriage my wife has taken care of the house, taken care of the children, taken care of me, and taken care of both of her parents. Now it is my turn to take care of her. She no longer knows who I am and will ask what I am doing in her house. But I truly believe that people with dementia have very short flashbacks so that just for an instant several times each day they do have a recollection of how things are and how things were.

Being a caregiver is a demanding task and I am grateful that I have been able to care for my Sweetheart. I have no regrets on the care that she was given. She has been a hospice patient for 4 years 10 months and 5 days. That much longevity as a hospice patient is almost unheard of. I know the care given and staying in her own home environment were great contributors to that longevity. My Sweetheart is now in a better place with a perfect mind and body. I know that sometime in the future we will have a grand reunion. I look forward to that day.

CHAPTER 1

The Beginning

I n the beginning God created the heaven and the earth. And the earth was without form, and void; and darkness was upon the face of the deep. And the Spirit of God moved upon the face of the waters. And God said, Let there be light; and there was light. And God saw the light, that it was good: and God divided the light from the darkness. And God called the light Day, and the darkness he called Night. And the evening and the morning were the first day. *Genesis 1:1-5.*

Our beginning was over 60 years ago in a small town in the West. It was a small farming town and each town at that time had at least one drug store. In each drug store was a soda fountain. I saw her sitting on a stool at the soda fountain with one of her boyfriends. She was a popular girl and always had a boyfriend or two or three. She was a member of the local high school pep club, the homemaking club, and was the homecoming queen at her high school during her senior year. She was raised on a family farm with two older sisters and one younger brother. She was the girl who most frequently helped her father doing the farm work.

I was raised on a family farm as well, in a neighboring small town. I had two older brothers, one younger sister, and one younger brother. There were enough boys in our family to help our father with the farm work. In addition to farming, we had livestock and a band of sheep. It was a good life growing up in that area at that time.

We danced. There was a movie theater where they changed the movie usually weekly. Things were different then. There was no television, no pizza parlors, no computers, no cell phones and no indoor plumbing. We danced. There was always a Saturday night dance at the local National Guard Armory and a small nearby college often had dances on Friday nights. If you had a date, you went to the dance. If you didn't have a date, you went to the dance. There were always lots of "stag" girls and boys at each dance. When you found someone of interest, you asked if you could take them home. That is how romances began and ours was no different. That was a long time ago.

She had regular medical check-ups and all of the normal tests recommended by the medical community. I would take her to the doctor and sit in the waiting room until she was finished. One day, the nurse said I needed to come and hear what the doctor was saying because my wife didn't think she could remember. From that time forward, I have always been present for the entire doctor visit. During one visit, the internal medicine doctor indicated that she should see a Neurologist and gave us a referral. At the conclusion of that visit, we were informed that she had DEMENTIA with Alzheimer's symptoms. Medications were prescribed and the Neurologist indicated that I must assume full responsibility for all medications. In addition, she indicated that I needed to acquire a copy of the book, "The 36 Hour Day" (A Family Guide to caring for people who have Alzheimer's Disease, Related Dementias, and Memory Loss) and read it. I did! It was very informative and was definitely a great help.

It isn't an easy task to take over something that your spouse has always done for herself. They become very defensive and wonder why you are taking their responsibilities away. They don't think they need your help and many times they don't. But then, there are the times when they need your help and they don't know it. Sometimes it is the simple things. She forgot to turn off the shower and it has been running and you're not sure how long. I try to remember that she is doing the best she can and above all, keep a good sense of humor.

She always took care of the check book. I made the money and she paid the bills. Everything was always paid on time and each month the check book was balanced to the penny. The one problem that I had with her was she embezzled—from me. You could never tell how much money was in the account by looking at the check book. She always had some money set aside and only she knew how much. That was OK though. I didn't complain. One day she told me that we had a problem and that she didn't have any coupons left to make house payments. I told her to call the finance company and tell them to send more. When she called, they told her she didn't need any coupons because the house was paid in full. She had been making double payments without my knowledge.

There came a day when she could no longer manage the checkbook. When she would see me doing something with the checkbook, she would always complain that I was taking away the things she had always done. I would try to assure her that it was not the case and that she just could no longer do that task and it wasn't her fault. That really didn't help. I soon realized that when I needed to do something with the checkbook, I needed to take things to a room so she couldn't see what I was doing. That certainly helped relieve the stress on both of us.

This past year, all of our family was together for Thanksgiving. It was a good time and although she couldn't tell you the name of anyone, she knew that they were family. Shortly after everyone had returned to their homes, I noticed that the TV remote control was missing for one of the sets. I searched the house over and was unable to find anything. I ordered a new remote control and when it arrived, I completed the reprogramming and was back in business. A few days later, I found the missing remote control in her dresser drawer. Now, the remote control for the family room TV is missing. I unsuccessfully searched the house but that is OK because I had a spare to reprogram. I still have a spare but I just don't know where to find it.

I am a full time Caregiver. It didn't start that way but over time has evolved to full time. That doesn't mean 8-5, five days a week. It means 24 hours a day and seven days a week, whatever and whenever required. Most of us sometime in our lives will be caregivers to someone. My Sweetheart has been a caregiver several times and I don't mean caring for our children. Twenty five years ago, her parents moved into our home. They were no longer able to care for themselves with one being legally blind and the other a severe diabetic. That was the beginning of a ten year care giving responsibility that she shouldered. Both lived the remainder of their lives in our home. Caring for them became more and more demanding as the years passed. We would tell people that we could go anyplace at any time but couldn't be away for more than an hour and a half. At one time during a doctor visit for her Mother, the doctor asked if it wasn't about time that she put her Mother in a nursing home. To that question, she responded "no it isn't time but if it ever comes, I'll know it". The time never came and her Mother was able to live out her life in our home.

We husbands don't really pay attention sometimes to the things that we should. We take for granted many things because our wives have always had that responsibility. When she can no longer shoulder that responsibility and it falls upon us, we just don't know what to do or how to do it. That gets even more pronounced when you think about personal things that they need to do but can no longer do for themselves. How often should she wash her hair? Can you blow dry her hair and make it look presentable? Can you cut and file her fingernails and toenails? The list goes on and on. It seems that there are new challenges every day. Just when we think we have everything figured out and under control, we find something new. Hopefully, as time goes on, we learn some of the tricks of the trade that makes life better for both of us.

When I was growing up, the term "stress" was not in the medical vocabulary. I'm convinced the term was used as a marketing tool to increase the business of some psychologist. The term gained momentum and is now widely used and treated. In my day they just told you to stop worrying. The same thing applies to death. When someone died, the mortician was called, there was a funeral service of some kind, and they were buried. Today when someone dies, they call the mortician, have and funeral service, bury them and then call in the grief counselors so they can assist them in healing. What is healing? The person died and is buried. Why do you need a person to help you grieve? Grief is a natural part of the process when someone dies. When my Sweetheart is no longer with us, it will be a sad day but not a day for a grief counselor. I have far too many fond memories and she will no longer be suffering from her affliction.

Strawberry Jam! Strawberry jam has become a silver bullet for getting her to eat. I like strawberry jam, the frozen kind. I have become an expert in making frozen strawberry jam. She may not have any appetite at all but I can give her a piece of toast covered with strawberry jam and she will eat every bite. I fixed her some scrambled eggs and ham along with a piece of toast and jam. She took one bite of the eggs and said she wasn't hungry. I put a little strawberry jam on the eggs and she ate every bite.

I have learned that when you are cooking, you need to guard your recipes carefully. You lay a spoon down, she will pick it up and wash it. You lay the recipe down, she will pick it up and put it away. The problem is where? During Thanksgiving, our daughter-in-law was making dinner rolls. She didn't bring a copy of her recipe but remembered most of it and then called her Mother to fill in the blanks. Midway through the process, her recipe became missing. We looked and looked without success. A week after they returned home, I found the recipe. She had put it away in one of her recipe books.

The basement is my sanctuary. I believe that everyone needs a sanctuary. It is the place that I go when I need to blow off steam or work on my current project. I have to have a project of some type to keep me occupied and keep me thinking about something other than care giving. My first project was writing down some of my life experiences. As a boy and young man, I hunted big game and decided I should write down my hunting experiences for my sons and grandsons. Then, I decided to write down my fishing experiences then farming experiences, sheep experiences, work experiences and so forth. When I finished, I had written eleven chapters with pictures where appropriate. It ended up being about 120 pages. My next project was pictures. We had drawers full of pictures and I have placed them in albums with an album for each of our children. I'm not sure what the next project will be but rest assured there will be one.

We try to live our lives as normally as possible. We go places, do things and have a good time doing them. I started playing golf years ago. I never was a very good player but I enjoyed the game. I particularly enjoyed playing in golf tournaments where I could compete with other people of similar skill level. I just enjoyed the competition. I play just as well in competition as when I'm just playing for fun but that is not the case with a lot of players, they fall apart.

My Sweetheart decided that she was going to start playing about the time that she was diagnosed with dementia. She didn't hit the ball a great distance with her longest drive being less than 100 yards. I always played from the men's tee box but moved her up to about the 200 yard marker. That way, we could keep the pace and not slow down the play for anyone. She likes to play with pink golf balls and always guards them as if no more will ever be made. One day we were playing and a seagull swooped down and snatcher her ball. It was a sight to see. She was running down the fairway waving her golf club and shouting at the seagull. He finally dropped her ball. As dementia progressed, we would still play. Sometimes I would get her up to the hitting area and tell her to hit and she would say she didn't know what to do. I would T up the ball for her, hand her the club and she immediately knew how to stand, how to hold the club and how to hit the ball. I frequently took her with me to play in tournaments. She would complain but she would go and end up enjoying the day. We went to a tournament late in the year and when we arrived to play, the wind was howling and the temperatures were cold. I bundled her up with coats and blankets but it was still cold. We came by the clubhouse during the tournament and she wanted to sit in the car where it was warm. I agreed, put her in the car and told her to stay and that I would be back to check on her in a while. A half hour later, a golf cart approached where we were playing and she was in the cart with someone from the clubhouse. They said she was out wandering around looking for me and they were afraid she would wander away or get hurt. I never left her alone again.

It is cold and wintery today and we have snow on the ground. I have this internal alarm clock that goes off at 5 AM each day. I have tried to reset the internal clock without success. My Sweetheart normally goes to bed early and sleeps late. Last night she went to bed early, spent most of the night roaming around the house, and was out of bed at 5:30 AM. I have tried to get her to lie down and sleep but she just isn't interested. I'm not sure what to expect for the remainder of the day but I'm sure it will be the unexpected.

I recall a story an older gentleman in our office told of his experiences in WW II. He was captured by the enemy and placed in a concentration camp where he stayed for several years. When the camp was liberated, the gates were thrown open and the prisoners rushed out onto the hillsides looking for food. Some allied planes flew over the area and were loaded with cases of food which they tossed out. Prisoners were running trying to get to the food and in the process a case of food struck a prisoner and he was decapitated. The older gentleman went on to say that some people thought the case of food that struck him was peaches and some thought it was tomatoes but that he never really did find out. Did it make a difference?

I frequently read in the newspapers extensive articles about Alzheimer's disease and other related dementias. Does my Sweetheart have Alzheimer's? I don't know but her doctor has said she has Alzheimer's symptoms. Does it make a difference? I say that it is kind of like the peaches and tomatoes. It doesn't really matter.

Sometimes she is cooperative and sometimes she resists everything I try to do. I've learned a few things that work for me. Never give the medicine while she is standing near a sink or toilet because it makes it too easy for her to throw it away. I had just gotten a new medication for her to try and had a 30 day supply. The first day when I gave her the capsule, she was standing near the toilet. She took the capsule and drank some water. I turned my back and she flushed the toilet. When I looked back, I noticed the capsule swirling around in the toilet. Now I only have a 29 day supply.

Personal hygiene can be a problem at times. I have always insisted that she shower each morning. Most of the time this is not a problem but on some occasions she just refused to shower. I can coax, plead, insist, and shout but it makes no difference, she just refuses. After several tries, sometimes I just give up and accept the fact that there will be no shower today. What happens tomorrow and the next if she refused? I just keep coaxing, pleading and insisting, shouting does no good. Rarely does this happen but it does happen. The same thing happens with the medications but I have always been successful in getting her to take them. However, I keep a pill grinder on hand in the event that I have to use alternative means.

I remember when my own Mother was in her mid 90's and we would go to visit. Often we would be sitting in the room with her visiting and she would look at me and say, "are you one of mine"? "Did you have any kids?" We often laughed about that but now it is not nearly as humorous. Several times each day my Sweetheart will look at me and ask "who are you?" She will go on to say things like: "What is your name; I have a husband but I don't know where he is now; where do you live?" The thing that I try to remember is that she is doing the best that she can. I can't imagine how frustrating it may be for someone who can't remember someone that they have lived with for over half a century.

I heard a story a short time ago about an older gentleman who was visiting his doctor. Things were running a little late and the older gentleman was getting quite nervous. The nurse asked him if there was a problem and he replied that he needed to be at the nursing home to visit his wife. The nurse responded that she was sure his wife really looked forward to his visits. He told her that his wife really didn't know he was there because she hadn't recognized him for years. To this the nurse responded that he shouldn't be nervous about being there at a certain time if she didn't remember him. He responded that she may not remember me but I sure remember her.

We just started a new medication that was prescribed to hopefully make her more cooperative. It is a tiny tablet to be taken once or twice a day. I started with twice a day and immediately dropped back to once a day. She became very nervous and anxious. I likened her to the Ever Ready Battery Bunny, she just didn't run down. She would jabber incoherently at times. Finally, she wouldn't sleep. She was up and roaming the house all night and consequently, I didn't sleep. Two nights in a row, no sleep for either of us. The nights were long. I stopped the pills and that night, we both slept a good long and restful sleep.

A distant relative who was a doctor said that in his earlier years that he thought that he was a good doctor. In his later years he determined that he was not nearly as good as he'd thought. He went on to say that now I listen to what my patients tell me and now I think that I am a good doctor. In the case of my own doctor, I recently had an episode with shingles. About 6 months later, I believed that I was having a recurrence. I went to my doctor's office and told the staff that I needed to see my doctor because I believed that I may have the shingles. They told me that it would be at least two weeks until I could see him. I went on to tell them that previously I was informed that it was important to see a doctor within 48 hours of a shingles episode and if my doctor was not available that I would find another. They immediately told me that I could have an appointment the next day. When I went for the appointment, the staff informed me that I would not see my doctor but would see another—was that OK? My response was, what choice do I have? If you can't see your primary care doctor when you need to, why have one.

My Sweetheart's doctor has said that when you need to see me and have no scheduled appointment, contact my nurse and we will work something out. Time after time, she has made her time available when she was needed. I have sent her emails through a special medical records web site and have had answers within a few hours. I even received an answer concerning a medical issue on New Year's Day. It makes it difficult for a doctor to listen to her patients when the patient can't remember the problem. At times they will wince with pain from some ailment and when you asked about the pain, they can't remember. A caregiver often must be the eyes, ears and mouthpiece for the patient. When issues arise, I try to keep some kind of daily medical diary so I can review the notes and give the doctor accurate information. I'm not sure the daily medical diary is the best way to keep track of information but it works for me. Some people just use a calendar where they can make notes and that works for them.

I worked for years with a good friend whose Mother-in-Law was afflicted with Multiple Sclerosis. As the years passed, the disease kept taking its toll. It wasn't long until she had no mobility except for a small electric scooter. She had a small home and was able to manage quite well but when special occasions arrived, it was often necessary to transport her and her scooter to other locations. Lacking a modern van with lift capability, my friend would hook his horse trailer to his pickup truck, load his Mother-in-Law into the horse trailer on her scooter, place a lawn chair beside the scooter for his wife, and proceed to the location. I'm sure you can imagine the scolding he would get if he traveled too fast or hit too many bumps in the road. But, the horse trailer worked for them. In today's environment he would be arrested for abuse of the elderly.

In 2006 we decided it was time to buy a new car. We had two cars and decided that we would become a one car family. We bought a big Lincoln Town Car and after my Sweetheart had driven it a few times, she said she didn't like it and wanted her own car, a smaller two door. We found one that she liked and bought it. A little over a year later, my Sweetheart was driving and pulled into a left turn lane behind a large van. The van was signaling and when it was clear, it made a left turn. My Sweetheart followed without regard to the oncoming traffic. We avoided a serious accident only because of the driving skills of the oncoming car. That day was the last day that she has driven. I didn't tell her she couldn't drive but made sure that she didn't. Today, some six years later, that car sits in our garage with 6400 miles on the odometer and still has the new car smell. Although she has stopped driving, she still has a set of car keys in her purse. The time is not yet right to dispose of the car.

I remember my own Mother and her automobile. When she was about 85, she called me and asked if I thought she was crazy if she bought a new car. I told her no, if she wanted a new car that she had 3 sons and one daughter living within 2 miles of her home and one of them would be glad to help her. She said she didn't want them to help her but she wanted me. We drove the 300 miles to her home the next weekend. We found a car that was nice and was equipped the way she wanted. It was a holdover model from the previous year and I told her that we could buy it for a very good price. She said she didn't like that car because it wasn't sporty enough for her. We bought the car she wanted and she drove for several years. Her trips were short and usually no more than 10 miles. One day she decided that she no longer felt safe driving and when she wanted to go someplace, she would contact someone and ask them to come and drive her using her car. That still gave her a feeling of independence. One day my sister called and said that one of her children was in need of a car and would like to buy my Mother's. I told her no, the time was not right. She kept the car for a few more years and then the time was right.

Paper napkins, paper towels, kleenex and anything else you can think of seems to get the attention of my Sweetheart. She folds them neatly and stacks them up. She places them in coat pockets, drawers, cupboards and anyplace she can think of. I am constantly throwing them away and she is constantly generating more. Frequently, she will take important papers and put them where she thinks they belong and then, of course, she doesn't remember where. I buy "forever" stamps and today I needed one. They are nowhere to be found. They are apparently a casualty to her fixation with papers. I have searched all of the common hiding spots and am convinced she has some secret spots that must be loaded with treasures.

I remember when I was working and a serious issue would arise which we totally disagreed with. Sometimes we would resist and pursue the issue in an effort to generate change. When we did pursue the issue, we realized that if we failed there could be some serious consequences. I would tell my people that if you want to cross the gorge to fight the dragon and rescue the maiden, be very sure that the maiden is worth rescuing. So it goes with care giving, many times issues or circumstances arise where we get frustrated with the way things are being done. We may insist that the person we are caring for do things a certain way or at a certain time. Does it really make a difference how it is done or when it is done? Most times it doesn't and we just end up extremely frustrated for no reason at all.

When my Sweetheart was ready for bed one evening, I noticed something unusual. She had the tops to her underwear on over her bra. I didn't think that much about it at the time but then I found out that she actually had 3 pair of underwear tops on at the same time. No harm done.

She had a birthday this past week. Birthdays don't mean that much anymore to most of us and she is no exception. However, there was an incident which I will always remember. One of our sons had taken us to dinner at a local restaurant. Several times during the dinner, she said she needed to go to the bathroom. I would escort her down a long hall to the ladies restroom and wait for her outside the door. The second trip, she came back outside of the restroom and said that she didn't go because she wasn't sure where she was supposed to go. She wanted me to come into the ladies room with her. Naturally, I declined. I pushed the door open for her to go inside and told her to just walk straight ahead to a vacant stall. She was unsure what to do and I kept giving her instructions with the door about half open. Thank goodness I could not see any other women in the room. Midway through me giving her instructions, one of the waiters came by and immediately told me that I couldn't go inside because that was for ladies only and I would have to use the one marked for men. I hurriedly explained to him that my wife had dementia and I was just trying to give her instructions.

Recently, we went to a local restaurant and she needed to visit the ladies room. She was escorted to the back of the restaurant and went inside the restroom. Immediately after she entered the room, an older lady approached and asked if she needed any assistance and that she could help if needed. She was thanked and just a few minutes after, another older lady approached and asked if I wanted her to check and make sure she was doing OK. In all of the times that she has been escorted to a ladies room, no one has ever offered their assistance and on that day there were two ladies that offered. The world is not such a bad place.

In addition to dementia, she also has arthritis in her right hip. It seems that she is in constant pain. The orthopedic doctor has told us that the only way to relieve the pain is by hip replacement surgery. In her state of mind, I have insisted that the surgery is not a viable option. Instead, we have been using different pain medications attempting to find one that is effective. Some that we have tried were effective for the pain but caused a great deal of confusion and anxiety.

My Sweetheart, like most of us, is a creature of habit. When she gets into bed, she always does it the same way. She places her right knee on the bed and then crawls onto the bed on her hands and knees. This puts a great deal of strain on her right hip which exacerbates the pain. I have repeatedly encouraged her to do differently with no success. Our bed is a high one. First, I made a ramp where she could walk up and sit on the edge of the bed and just roll over. She didn't like that so I made a step. That didn't work. The latest, we decided to lower the height of the bed. One of our sons has a demolition saw and we just cut the legs off about twelve inches shorter. Now she can easily get into bed without crawling on her hands and knees. She is a creature of habit and just keeps crawling.

Today is a bitter cold day. I need to put lots of clothing on her when I take her outside for any reason. The problem is, when she gets cold she knows something isn't right but really can't tell you she is cold. As I look back over the last few months, many things have changed and none were for the best. She was helping me make a bed this morning and needed to put a pillow slip on the pillow. She just didn't know how. I could tell her what to do but she just didn't understand. Words have very little if any meaning for her. She can still read a word or two but has no idea what she is reading. I'm sure that is the way things are when she hears someone talking. It just doesn't make any sense. When she talks it sometimes doesn't make sense. I will ask her what she just said and her response will be that she doesn't know because she can't remember. That becomes so frustrating for me as a caregiver but, I can't imagine how frustrating it is for her. That makes it especially difficult for a doctor to treat a patient if the patient can't really talk sense and make the doctor understand the problem.

Sometimes the days seem long and the nights seem short but that is life. Although things get quite trying and demanding at times, there are many good times and I will have many good memories. I will cherish these times above all others.

And thus ended the first day.

CHAPTER 2

The Second Day

And God said, Let there be a firmament in the midst of the waters, and let it divide the waters from the waters. And God made the firmament, and divided the waters which were under the firmament from the waters which were above the firmament: and it was so. Genesis 1:6-7.

I was awakened about 11 PM with the bedroom lights on and she was standing over me asking my name and what I was doing in her house? This was not an unusual occurrence. In fact it happens quite frequently. What can one do about it? Nothing. It just happens and a person has to learn to live with it. I just can't imagine what is going through her mind and the confusion that she must feel. From my side, I feel confused also and really quite hurt that she doesn't remember me whom she has lived with for over 50 years. She is doing the best that she can and I must always remember that.

I am trying various things to cope with the issue of her getting up around midnight and roaming the house. It occurred again and I decided that I would get out of bed and do something constructive. I was working on my income taxes on the computer when she came in all dressed up and ready to go someplace, not sure where, but someplace. She didn't know why she had dressed. I was able to get her back into bed and then watched TV for a short time. She then went to sleep and seemed to sleep well. Another approach is definitely needed to cope with this problem.

It is now 2:15 AM and no sleep at all tonight. We have been struggling with the pain in her right hip and two days ago she had a hip injection. Midafternoon of that day, she laid on the bed and napped. The nap turned into a sixteen hour sleep. I was unable to awaken her for medications or to prepare her for bed. She just slept in her regular clothing to include her eye glasses. During the day following the big sleep, she was very uncooperative, refusing to take some of her medications and refusing to shower. She did remove her blouse and put on a clean one. She didn't like the trousers she was wearing and put on a second pair. Early in the evening I was successful in getting her clothing removed and getting her into pajamas. I felt like that was a great victory. Then, the marathon began. She would straighten the bed, get into the bed, get out of the bed, wander around the house turning on all of the lights, turn off all of the lights and start over again. It has now been like that for hours. Finally, I just gave up. I'm paying the price now for the big sleep. What is she doing now? I haven't a clue but you can rest assured that it isn't sleeping. Did the hip injection help? It is too soon to tell. It is difficult caring for someone with dementia and when that is coupled with another ailment, the problems are just compounded.

I have come to the conclusion that the reason she will put on two trousers at times or two tops at times is my fault. Before her dementia had progressed, she always had several pair of trousers and several tops all neatly folded and sitting on a bench at the foot of the bed. I have gradually reduced the size of those piles but still have about three trousers and three tops. I have concluded that if she doesn't see those extra items of clothing readily available that she won't go looking for them. I'm reducing those items to zero and putting everything on hangers or in drawers so they are out of sight. Hopefully this will make life a little easier for both of us.

I have a bottle with a slotted plastic lid where I put my loose change. When the bottle becomes full, I separate the coins and stack them into stacks of 10 and put them in coin rolls. She watched and decided she wanted to help. She carefully counted out 10 coins in one area of the table. Then, she counted them again, and again, and again. Finally, she left the table and went to another room until I was done. All of the time I kept encouraging her but she just disregarded the encouragement. Some days she can count very well. Some days she can read words but they don't appear to have any meaning to her. She likes to clean and straighten the bed. I encourage her to do all that she can and praise her for her efforts. I don't know if it helps her but I will continue to praise her because it helps me.

About two years ago, my Sweetheart could still remember things quite well and understood what was happening. We attended a seminar on estate planning that was sponsored by a high priced attorney. The seminar was very enlightening and we determined that we needed to establish a family trust. We then attended a free consultation with that same lawyer and she looked at our information and outlined to us what she believed that we needed. She also quota a price for her services and it was quite expensive. When I hesitated to accept, she started to apply the pressure. I informed her that I would never spend that much money without giving it more thought and study. The next day, a flyer from a local attorney came with our newspaper which offered the same kinds of documents for less than one-third. Needless to say, we didn't return to the more expensive attorney. All of our assets were converted to a family trust and we each have a will, a living will, and a power of attorney. We made copies of all of the documents and gave a set of them to each of our children. It was timely for us to take that action. Have you taken care your estate planning? If you haven't, don't wait too long.

For several years, we have talked about funeral arrangements for when we pass on. Final arrangements can be trying for survivors so we decided to make our own arrangements while we were living. We now have established pre-paid funerals for each of us. We have selected the cemetery and made the necessary arrangement. We have picked our caskets, prepared draft funeral programs, and also prepared draft obituaries. Here again, we made copies of the funeral arrangement documents and furnished them to our children. We should have started this process sooner as my Sweetheart couldn't contribute much to the process. However, we had discussed most of the issues at various times and I was comfortable knowing her wishes.

Pajamas have become a significant issue at times. When bed time comes, I always want her to put on her pajamas. For some reason she seems to always resist. I beg, I plead, I insist and she still resists. Sometimes I just give up and tell her to sleep in her clothing. I have found that if I lay out her pajamas and then put on my pajamas that she will follow suit. When I arise each morning, I remove my pajamas and lay them over a railing, put on my clothing and retire to our basement. One morning after a particular bad night, I followed the same routine. When I came upstairs a few hours later, she had arose and was dressed. She had a different pair of trousers which I did not recognize but assumed that she had gotten them from the closet. That evening when it was pajama time, I laid out her pajamas and went to get mine. It was then that I realized the trousers she was wearing were actually my pajama bottoms. They surely looked much nicer on her than they did on me.

She has always been extremely concerned about her appearance. She wanted her clothing to look nice and put on a reasonable amount of makeup. She didn't overdo the makeup but was really quite conservative in the application. She had lots of eye liner pencils, mascara brushes, lipstick, and eye makeup. With her no longer able to do much except apply lipstick, it became my responsibility to worry about makeup. I really didn't worry about it and believed she really didn't need to worry about it either. As a result it was just lipstick which she could apply. I disposed of all of the other makeup as it was not essential and would only make her confused. One morning something popped into her head about makeup. She decided that she wanted to put on some eye makeup. When I came into the bedroom, she was intently applying lipstick to her eye lids. I explained to her that you didn't use lipstick on your eye lids. I looked around and found some eye makeup but the urge had passed and she was no longer interested.

She has three pair of glasses. They are somewhere but I don't have any idea where. A few nights ago, we were lying in bed and she was wearing her glasses. I told her that I would put them on the dresser. She said no, she would just put them on the night stand at the side of the bed. The next morning she said she needed her glasses. I started looking and none of her glasses were anyplace to be found. I have searched the bedroom and various other rooms of the house without success. They must be with the TV remote control or in some other location which surely is loaded with treasures. Several days later, I found the glasses in the Kleenex box, under all of the Kleenexes.

Shoes have become a serious issue at times. A short time ago, along towards evening, I noticed that she had shoes with buckles which were both on the inside of her ankle. When I looked more closely, the shoes were not a matching pair and one was on the wrong foot. Following that incident, I paid more attention to her shoes. It wasn't long until I noticed a similar situation but was able to get it corrected. After that, I filled three bags with shoes which had straps and put them in our storage room. She still has too many shoes and I need to remove some additional pairs. Too many choices just adds to the confusion.

There are times when she seems quite helpless and there are times when she seems to be quite independent. Many times she needs help to do everything but then times when she doesn't want any help at all. I have never found a pattern as to why this happens and I'm convinced that there is no pattern. I just have to take things one day at a time and sometimes, one hour at a time.

People have been telling me for some time that I need to get some help and get away from things periodically. I have listened and agreed but didn't really believe them. I'm beginning to realize that I do need some help. I need to have some "my time" periodically to get away and let my head clear. I have decided that I'm going to try to find a person who can come into our home for 7 hours a day for 2 days each week. I'll just get away and do something relaxing or fun for me.

My Sweetheart has difficulty walking due to the arthritis in her right hip. When we go to the grocery store, she refuses to ride in a wheel chair and can't navigate on one of the electric carts for the handicapped. We just move along very slowly. I have to keep a constant watch because she will wander away. She likes to talk to people and especially small children. She will walk out of her way to talk with the kids. Also, it becomes a problem when she walks up to another grocery cart and starts rummaging through the groceries. I frequently have to explain to other shoppers that she just doesn't realize what she is doing. They all seem to take it well but don't have much choice. I'm sure that we will meet someone someday who will become angry or really offended. So be it. She needs to get out of the house periodically.

She still has concerns about her appearance. She will go to the closets and take out clothing and change clothes. She rarely replaces the clothing in the closets. I make a constant effort to replace them as soon as possible. She recently was looking at jackets in the entry coat closet. She didn't like the color of the trousers she was wearing when she put on one of the coats. She immediately removed her trousers while standing in the entry way. Thank goodness we did not have any visitors at the time. When I told her that she needed to put on some trousers, she immediately went to the bedroom and put on the trousers that she had remove.

Now she is putting the used toilet tissue in the trash can close to the toilet rather than in the toilet. I have repeatedly tried to make her understand that the trash can is not the proper place. She always agrees with me but never changes. I've decided that rather than make an issue that I just need to empty the trash can more often. I believe I may be getting a little smarter. Rather than getting upset or making issues out of small things, I've just decided that it isn't worth the anguish. I recently read a short quote that is very appropriate: "Wouldn't it be wonderful if when we lost our temper, we never found it again."

She can no longer open a car door or put on a seat belt because she doesn't remember how it is done. The doors to our home have a lock on the door knob and also a dead bolt. She has great difficulty opening the doors. Each time that I go outside to pick up the mail or retrieve my newspaper, I'm fearful that she will inadvertently lock the door. I have a spare house key in my garage and two ways that I can gain entry to the garage in the event the doors are locked. Frequently when she needs to visit the bathroom, she will ask me to take her because she doesn't remember where it is located in our home. She frequently is unable to turn off the shower water—but she always remembers to dry the shower door. She can't fix anything to eat but she always keeps the kitchen clean and when I am cooking, every utensil that I lay down will be immediately scooped up, washed, dried and then she looks for the place to put it. She will always put it someplace but there is neither rhyme nor reason for some of the places where things are found at a later time.

I recently ordered a two shelf bookcase. When it arrived, of course, it had to be assembled. I gathered the necessary tools and began the task. When I needed to refer to the instructions, they were missing. Of course, she didn't know anything about their whereabouts. I later found them in one of her favorite hiding spots. It wasn't long until I was missing one of my tools. I soon was able to locate that and continue the work. Between looking for the assembly instructions, looking for my tools and doing the actual work, the task was extended long past what I had expected. One of my tools was not found until the following day.

I contacted a family friend who has lived in our area for years and whose profession was in nursing. I wanted to question her on what could be done to better care for my Sweetheart. One suggestion that was made was to secure a four wheeled walker (the kind with hand brakes and a seat). I immediately told her that the walker would be un-usable because my Sweetheart wouldn't be able to master the hand brakes. She said that when she cared for her mother in her home, she used the four wheeled walker extensively, not as a walker but as a people mover. She would seat her mother and then drag the walker all over the house. It was much more maneuverable than a wheel chair especially in older homes.

Buttons, snaps and zippers in her trousers seem to be more and more of a problem for her. We went to a local clothing store in an effort to find trousers which had an elastic waist. We were told by one of the customers that the Alfred Dunner brand of clothing was that type and was stocked by J. C. Penney's. We visited the local store and found what we wanted. They had a wide variety of sizes. We found the correct size and length so it was not necessary to have them altered. Those types of trousers will work much better than those with buttons, snaps or zippers.

We are always struggling with the appetite. She just refuses to eat and will only take a few bites and then says that she is full. I coax and plead but always give up. She doesn't have the sense of taste but has always enjoyed sweet or tarty foods. I try to have some of those available at all times. I gave her one of the small ice cream cones and she ate just a few bites and then started to wrap it in a napkin to put away until she wanted more. I told her that it needed to be put in the freezer or it would melt. She wouldn't listen and kept wrapping it. I left the kitchen and came back in just a few minutes to retrieve the ice cream cone and place it in the freezer. It was no place to be found. She doesn't remember where she put it and I have not been successful in finding it. Someday I will and I hate to think where.

My brother's wife was a victim of dementia. She had put her rings someplace and they had no idea where. I'm not sure if they have ever found them. I decided that I needed to do something with her good rings. I think I have all of them and have placed them inside a pouch and now they are in our safety deposit box. I'm sure that she has some other jewelry which should be there also and one day I will make it happen.

Pajamas are a problem again. She refused to remove her clothing and put on the pajamas at bedtime. Most recently, she went to sleep in her clothing so I just covered her with a blanket and left her lying on top of the bed. Sometime during the night she arose, removed her clothing and got into bed without pajamas. Then, early in the morning, she decided she needed pajamas and put on the tops of one pair and the bottoms of another. Really none of this made any difference. She could have just slept in her clothing, without clothing, or with pajamas. The important thing was that she slept well. I really didn't get too concerned about anything but did find it quite humorous.

We went to the grocery store and I put her in our wheel chair. I pushed the wheel chair with one hand and carried groceries in a hand held grocery basket with the other hand. There is a normal traffic pattern in most all grocery stores and this one was no different. The problem was that the heavy items were deposited in the basket at the beginning of the visit and the lighter items at the end. By the time we arrived at the check stand, I was completely tired out. My idea of grocery shopping that way was not a good one. I think in the future that I will definitely do my grocery shopping differently.

The problem with loss of appetite seems to get worse as time goes on. I keep trying different things but haven't really found anything that seems to work for the long term. The latest effort is back again with strawberries. I wash them, remove the stems, place them in a blender and essentially liquefy them, add sugar and lemon juice. I give her about 1/3 of a glass mixed with 2/3 of a glass of orange/pineapple juice. She seems to enjoy that and will drink several glasses each day. I have tried Ensure and similar products without success.

About 6 weeks ago my Sweetheart had a right hip injection. Now when she walks you can hear her coming with a crunching and grinding of bone on bone. We went for a regular doctor's visit and as usual, the doctor asked how are things going? I told her that I wouldn't answer that until she walked my Sweetheart across the room and back and sat her down. She walked her part way across the room, sat her down and asked if we were prepared to talk about hospice. My response was that subject was on my list. We were then referred to a local hospice and were contacted a short time after returning home. The nurse came with the require papers and also performed her initial evaluation. During the evaluation, the nurse attempted to get a blood pressure reading. She was unsuccessful but as time wore on, just as she was leaving, she was able to get a good blood pressure reading. The following day, a nurse's aide (CNA) came to take care of showering and to trim finger and toe nails. She was unsuccessful and left without accomplishing any of her tasks. I'm sure it will be necessary to administer some sort of sedative, at least initially, for them to be able to perform their services. They each plan to visit two times a week on different days. I am certainly looking forward to the program and I'm sure it will be a great benefit for us both.

We have a small stand-up shower stall and a bathtub with a shower. On the initial visit from hospice, I told the nurse that I intended buying a shower nozzle with a flexible hose and replace the fixed shower head over the bathtub. When the CNA made her initial visit, I showed her the flexible hose shower head. Her response was that it would be better for now in the stand-up shower because she could then stand in the shower doorway and direct the spray as she needed. In the past when I provided shower assistance, I stood on a stool outside the shower door and gave instructions while looking over the top of the door. The flexible hose shower head works much better and now I can give hands-on assistance when needed. I'm sure there will be many more tricks to the trade that can be learned from observing and questioning the hospice people.

It is hard to figure out the rationale sometimes when we receive prescription medications. Along with the dementia, we are confronted with the problems associated with severe arthritis in the right hip. When she walks, you can hear her coming as the hip bones grind and click. The pain medication which provides the most relief has a dosage of 1-2 tablets every 4 hours as needed for pain. The next prescription for the same medication indicated a dosage of 1-2 tablets every 6 hours as needed for pain. I have been experimenting with the dosage to find what works best for my Sweetheart. I've tried all different time and dosage combinations. Our prescriptions for pain are furnished through a mail order pharmacy where we order a 90 day supply each time. A short time ago I placed an order and received only 240 tables for the 90 day supply. When I questioned them about the quantity, I was told that they had contacted the doctor and he had told them to send that amount. The doctor was contacted and a supplemental number was sent. It seems that the best pain control comes with giving 2 tablets every 6 hours given in the morning, noon and evening. When she wakes in the middle of the night with pain, I also give 2 tablets at that time making a daily dosage of 8 tablets or 720 tablets for a 90 day supply. A far cry from the 240 tablets we had initially received.

My Sweetheart can't really tell you much only sometimes she will say that her leg hurts. One morning I had great difficulty waking her. When I finally did get her awake, she was groggy, confused and incoherent. I decided that maybe she was overmedicated with the pain medication. I have now reduced the pain medications to one tablet 4 times each day. The first day seemed to go well but the sleep that first night wasn't that good. It may be necessary to adjust someplace in between so we can control the pain without causing an adverse effect on her sleep and cooperativeness.

She has never been a wanderer. I'm thankful for that. I have bought her a dementia necklace and also an ID bracelet so she would have some sort of identification. Both are casualties as I can no longer find where she put them. Recently I awoke in the middle of the night and it seemed cold. When I went exploring as to the cause, I found the front door was wide open. Also, the garage door was open, the lights in our kitchen, garage, and on our patio were burning brightly. Now I'm concerned that she may become a wanderer. I'm still trying to decide what I should do.

On several occasions, the hospice nurse has asked when the dementia was first noted. As one looks back over the years it becomes confusing as to when certain events happened. Some kind of landmark is needed to really identify events. Such is the case with identifying when dementia was first noted. In early 2003 we were asked by our church to do some volunteer work in one of our facilities. We worked one day each week and often substituted when other people needed time off. The tasks required fairly significant memorization. We enjoyed the work very much but in early 2005, my Sweetheart said she could no longer do that work because she just had so much trouble remembering how to perform her duties. We took a short leave of absence but decided in May 2005 that we should be released. Her memory has continued to deteriorate since that time.

Doctors are wonderful people. They are often placed on a pedestal and we think they have all of the answers. The problem is they don't. Mostly the reason they don't is because we just don't tell them the problems. They see the patient every few months and don't have any idea what the problems are unless we tell them. As a caregiver, we have the responsibility to be the eyes, the ears, and the mouthpiece for the patient. As dementia progresses, the patient becomes less and less able to communicate how they feel and where they have pain. We can only find out through observation and questioning. Hopefully we will be up to the challenge.

We try to get out of the house when we can and frequently go out for lunch. One of our sons who lives nearby is often available and meets us. As we were preparing to leave, my Sweetheart was in the process of trying to put on eye makeup. She had the tube of lipstick and was attempting to apply it to her eye lids. I was able to stop that before it was started but then we arrived at the restaurant, I noted that she had taken some eye liner and had painted one eyelid. I tried to remove it at the restaurant but she resisted so we had lunch with one eyelid painted and it was a good lunch. Sometimes when situations occur, we try to make a big issue over things that really don't make that much difference. We worry too much about what other people may think but who really cares.

We found a lady who does hair in her home. I take my Sweetheart to her about once each month for color, cut and style. Today was hair day. The color went fine but the shampoo was a disaster. During the process, I gave her ½ of a pill which should have a calming effect. It didn't work and only made her more confused and irritated. We finally were able to get the shampooing completed after thoroughly soaking her and the surrounding area. When it came time to dry her hair, the beautician said that I had to hold the drier because she wouldn't. Finally, we had to abandon our hair day efforts. Hopefully in a few days we will be able to return for the haircut and styling. It is my intention to shorten her hair significantly which will make it easier to manage, also, it may be necessary to forego the color in the future.

Last night was one of those nights. The hospice nurse had instructed me to give her one of the tablets that is prescribed to make her more cooperative. It was to be given the night before shower day so the medication would take effect but she would not be in a deep sleep at shower time. I followed the instructions and gave her the tablet about 8 PM. She never slowed down all night. She would get into bed, get out of bed, make the bed, tear the bed apart and make the bed again, put on her PJ's, take off her PJ's and generally just busied herself all night. Finally at 4 AM, I just gave up and got out of bed and dressed. What is she doing right now? I don't have a clue but I'm sure she is not sleeping. It will be interesting to see how the shower goes this morning. Also, in the afternoon, she is scheduled to have a haircut. Neither the shower nor the haircut happened.

After talking with the hospice CNA today, she suggested that I give her another of the medications and that maybe when they were in her system that they would be effective. I decided to give it a try but now it appears that was a bad decision. She has become essentially nonfunctional. Without the medication, she could at least understand some things but now she is just in a stupor. I finally did get her to the bathroom and now she is sleeping. Hopefully things won't turn into a disaster for tonight. I don't believe that we will use this new medication again anytime in the near future. Although at times she is uncooperative, that is still better than the state of affairs when she is given this new medication. A different pill or another pill is not always the best way to go.

It seems that the food that she eats really well is bread, chicken gravy and roasted chicken. I take ½ slice of bread and break it into small pieces, break the chicken into small pieces, and cover it with chicken gravy. Then, she washes that down with orange/pineapple juice which is spiked with fresh strawberries, sugar, and lemon juice which is blended. How long that she will continue to eat that is anyone's guess. I have also found that she really doesn't like cereal with milk but will eat something like Honey Smacks as just a snack. I have started keeping a small bowl on the kitchen cabinet so they are always in sight.

She has a great deal of difficulty walking with her bad hip. Today seems worse than normal and most of the day I have moved her around the house in a wheel chair. That works reasonably well but with a home that was constructed over 40 years ago, the hallways and doorways are narrow. They just don't lend themselves to movement in wheel chairs. A neighbor who is also a nurse by profession has said the 4 wheeled walkers with a seat works extremely well as a people mover especially in older homes where spaces are somewhat restricted. I intend to pursue that with the hospice people.

Restaurants are strange places at times. We frequently eat lunch in a restaurant because we need to eat and also need to get out of the house. Generally it is an enjoyable time. My Sweetheart and I always share a meal and prefer that the kitchen split the meal between two plates. Most restaurants are happy to split the meal but there are a few that just refuse. One particular restaurant informed us that they had a high tech kitchen and if they were to split our meal between two plates

26

that they would need to hire an additional person. Needless to say, we don't visit that restaurant any longer and have given them extensive adverse publicity.

We recently visited a restaurant and as usual, my Sweetheart needed to visit the bathroom. I escorted her to the bathroom and was waiting outside when one of the waitresses exited. She asked if I was waiting for the lady inside and that she seemed a little confused. When I told her that was who I was waiting for, she immediately returned to the bathroom to provide any assistance that was needed. She left the bathroom and in just a few minutes returned to see if additional assistance was needed. A few weeks later, we returned to that same restaurant and that same waitress remembered us and came to our table and offered further assistance if needed. Experiences of that nature restores ones faith in the younger generation.

Yesterday was not a good day – in fact it was terrible. I spent most of the day moving her around inside the house in a wheel chair. She just can't walk with the bad hip. We tried a new medication which was supposed to have a calming effect but it didn't. It only made bad matters worse. In addition, there was no sleep. We tried to get her into the shower but that didn't happen. We tried to give her a sponge bath but only got the feet and legs and then gave up. When it was bed time, she wouldn't get into bed but spent most of the night sitting on the side of the bed mumbling. Were there any bright spots? Yes, there was one and it was on her upper lip. Apparently when I was not looking, she opened a bottle of finger nail polish and painted an area above her upper lip with hot pink glossy polish. Needless to say, the finger nail polish has been removed using polish remover.

I believe we are entering a new chapter in her care. It may be time for a hospital bed, a ramp is needed to get her in and out of the house in a wheel chair, and a four wheeled walker with a seat is needed to move her around inside the house. One way or another, I need to make these things happen.

She won't take her medications. I have removed all of the over the counter medications, crushed the prescription medications and put them in a small amount of water but she won't drink. I crushed the prescription medications and put them in strawberry mix but she won't eat it so I added a small amount of juice which she won't drink. I'll just have to keep trying. She refuses to move and go to the bathroom or to have a shower. I have a conventional walker which maybe she could use but she won't try. It seems to be one of those won't days—won't eat, won't drink, won't take a shower, won't go to the bathroom and won't get dressed. We will see what the remainder of the day brings.

I have a new medication which is intended to let her rest and be more cooperative. I was instructed to give her one tablet each night. The first night when I gave her the tablet, she became very calm and began sleeping. She never awoke until 11 AM the following day. Then, she napped a little off and on. The next night I decided to only give her ½ of a tablet. That worked well for about one hour and then she became somewhat nervous so I gave her the other half of the tablet. Since that time she hasn't slept at all. She is up hobbling around, taking the bed apart, remaking and muttering. We now have a bedside commode which she hasn't used yet. I fastened a roll of toilet tissue to the side of the commode. She has spent most of the night tearing pieces of toilet tissue off the roll, folding them neatly and stacking them on her night stand. By morning, I'm sure the roll of toilet tissue will be gone, all folded neatly and stashed in various places around the bedroom. It is now 1:30 AM and I have given up all hope of getting any sleep tonight. I hope I am surprised when I return to the bedroom.

The hospice nurse delivered the materials to get a urine sample. I was sure that the process of getting a good sample would be an almost insurmountable task. A short time after the materials were delivered, she said she needed to use the bathroom. I immediately installed the "hat" to catch the sample and covered the toilet tissue so it was not in her view. A short time later, the sample had been collected and stored waiting for pickup.

Tonight appears to be one of those nights. She won't put on PJ's, she won't lay down, she just wants to wander. She was diagnosed today with a urinary tract infection. Now we are treating the infection, pain meds for the bad hip, and trying to cope with the dementia. Any one is enough at one time but we have three problems. She just sits on the side of the bed and mutters in a low voice. At times she will hobble over to the sink area in the master bedroom and rearrange items on the vanity, then back to sitting on the side of the bed. The night seems to get longer and longer.

It is the small things sometimes that one really notices where they have lost their ability to cope with everyday living. Today we were driving and she wanted a comb. We have several combs in a zip lock plastic bag in the glove box of our car. She had no problem finding the bag with the combs when she was told where to look. She did have a problem trying to get a comb out of the zip lock bag. Finally, I unzipped the bag, she took a comb but couldn't understand how to close the bag. She just didn't understand when I tried to tell her what to do. That really isn't a problem but just another indicator of her inability to function.

Wonders never cease! She took a shower somewhat willingly. I had placed a shower stool in the standup shower so that she wouldn't need to stand. I sprayed warm water on the shower stool but when she walked into the shower she said, without even testing, that the shower stool was cold. I placed a small hand towel over the stool and we proceeded without interruption.

After the shower, we went to a restaurant for lunch. Midway through the lunch, I was informed that she needed to visit the bathroom. I found the hostess and explained the problem. She talked to her manager and then accompanied us to the bathroom taking my wife inside to provide assistance. She immediately came back outside and said that I needed to go inside and assist her. She said she would be the gate guard. I went inside and provided the assistance and when we exited, the hostess was nowhere in sight. That experience could easily have ended in an embarrassing situation but thank goodness it didn't.

And thus ended the second day.

CHAPTER 3

The Third Day

A nd God said, Let the waters under the heaven be gathered together unto one place, and let the dry land appear: and it was so. And God called the dry land Earth; and the gathering together of the waters called the Seas: and God saw that it was good. And God said, Let the earth bring forth grass, the herb yielding seed, and the fruit tree yielding fruit after his kind, whose seed is in itself, upon the earth: and it was so. And the earth brought forth grass, and herb yielding seed after his kind, and the tree yielding fruit, whose seed was in itself, after his kind: and God saw that it was good. Genesis 1:9-12.

How long is a day? Everyone knows that answer, a day is 24 hours. How long is a night? I don't believe anyone knows that answer except a night can be very, very long. I gave up trying to sleep at 3 AM and decided that I should do something constructive. First, I vacuumed the basement and then I started doing some writing. A short time later, I heard a noise coming from upstairs and decided I should investigate. My Sweetheart was in the kitchen and was worried about the lighted numbers on the clock and the lighted dial on the control pad of our recliner. I escorted her to the bedroom where I found the bed had been completely torn apart and stacked in the middle with the pillows laying on the floor. The only thing left on the bed was the mattress cover and the mattress. She had removed several articles of clothing from the closet, taken them off the hangers and they were piled in a heap at the end of the bed. I've always believed that in the caregiver business, one must have a sense of humor. When I saw the mess in the bedroom, I could only smile as I worked making the bed and caring for the clothing. I kind of suspect that a person with dementia has very small flashbacks of reality. I also suspect my Sweetheart was smiling at times looking at me making the bed and cleaning up the mess.

This afternoon and evening were not good times. I was trying to do some outside work and kept going by the big windows and waiving. Soon she walked to the front door and was standing on the steps. I put her in the wheel chair and moved her to the work area but she refused to stay seated. I soon stopped working outside and brought her back inside where she could be seated. During the process, her hip almost failed and the pain became excruciating. She has always been a pain tolerant person. Some extra pain medication was given but it didn't seem to be effective. She had a great deal of trouble laying down on the bed and would cry with pain when she was laying down. When the pain would subside, she would say she needed to use the bathroom. By the time we could get her off the bed and onto the bedside commode, she would be in a great deal of pain and was unable to do anything. We would get her back onto the bed and start the process over again. The third time was finally the charm. I felt so sad and helpless for her and there was just nothing that I could do to make things any less painful. The pain medication finally started to take effect but now is the beginning of one of those long nights. Tomorrow I will place an order for a hospital bed which should make things easier getting her into and out of bed.

We have lived in the same home for over 42 years. The master bedroom has an adjoining bath and a large walk in closet. On the door of the walk in closet is a full length mirror. Last night as we lay in bed, she kept talking about the other people that were in the room. I finally realized that she was looking at the full length mirror and believed our reflection was other people. I attempted to explain that the figures she saw were only our reflection. Finally, it became necessary to tape a large towel over the reflective area so she could rest.

She is no longer mobile. She can stand but when trying to take a step, the leg on the right side buckles and she almost falls. There are times when she will take a few steps using a conventional walker but mostly it is just standing, sitting and laying. It becomes difficult to put her in a wheel chair unless there is a way to get the chair directly behind her. She just doesn't understand that she needs to turn as she sits. When she needs to use the bedside commode, I move the wheel chair up to a conventional walker and have her stand. Then the wheelchair is removed and the commode is placed directly behind her. Seldom does she understand any instructions which may be given. I repeat the instructions over and over again in an effort to make her understand. It is a frustrating process and certainly will not improve.

A short time ago, the hospice nurse asked if she could go to the bathroom by herself or if I needed to help her. She has a problem getting to the bathroom and getting onto the stool. That has now changed. The last time that I took her to the bathroom all went well until the end. I'm sure you have heard the saying, "the job isn't finished until the paperwork is done." It became very apparent that she just didn't know what to do or how to do it to finish the job by doing the paper work.

The appetite seems to be getting worse. Some of the old standbys are no longer working. Frozen strawberry jam does not seem to have any appeal to her and the orange/pineapple juice spiked with fresh strawberries just isn't working well any longer. This morning her total breakfast was two bites of home canned pears and a small amount of juice. She ate two bites of a spam sandwich and about two bites of jello with pineapple and two sips of juice for lunch. Dinner was about the same. I have unsuccessfully tried the special drinks like Ensure. Her weight loss during the last month was 13 pounds. The hospice people tell me that this is normally what can be expected but it is hard for me to accept.

The hospital bed has side rails to keep the patient in bed. The problem with the side rails is that they are only at the head of the bed. There have been constant problems with her sitting up on the side of the bed during the night and never laying down again unless assisted. We have a side rail that can be slid under the mattress and the side raised to further assist keeping people in bed. Last night the second side rail was installed so the railing extended the full length of the bed. During the night I awoke with her sitting on the side of the bed. The second side rail had somehow been removed and was laying on the floor, all of the sheets and blankets were also on the floor. Although her mind doesn't work well on most things, it seemed an easy task for her to dismantle all of my efforts.

I tried a different approach on the hospital bed. We have it sitting in the master bedroom with one side of the bed snug to the end of the master bed. I removed the side rail on the side by the master bed and installed it at the foot on the other side. Now I have side rails at both the head and foot on one side of the bed. The first night with that arrangement seemed to work well and she was unable to exit the bed during the night. Hopefully both of us will sleep better in the future.

I have tried various methods to help her understand and remember things. Small name tags with bold letters were made to identify items in drawers, names of people in pictures, and tasks needing to be performed. For example, one tag said "BRUSH YOUR TEETH" – "PUT ON DEODORANT". Those tags are now gone. They no longer have any meaning to her. She may, at times, be able to read a word or phrase but they are just words or phrases without any meaning.

Hospice ordered a lift and it was delivered today. There is not a lot of room in the master bedroom so use is rather restricted. It can be used to lift her into bed from a wheel chair and also out of bed into the wheel chair. That is definitely a plus and is very helpful.

We were standing by the vanity and she indicated that she needed something for her lips. She has quit using lipstick but routinely uses chap stick. I handed her a tube of chap stick with the lid removed. She immediately bit off the end and began chewing. In the past, she has also used mouth wash and a liquid for dry mouth. In both cases the solutions are not to be swallowed. We have now discontinued the use of those products because she automatically swallows the liquid without regard to instructions not to swallow.

What is a Gait/Transfer Belt? I had never heard of such a thing. The hospice people brought one and it is used to help lift a patient. It is a large webbed belt with a metal buckle. It is fastened around the patient just under the arms and is used when lifting them to a standing position or from a laying position. You just grasp the belt and pull. In other words, it gives you something to hang onto when lifting. It is a great addition and I also use it to keep her in the wheel chair when I don't want her standing. I simply put it around her and buckle it behind the back of the wheel chair. The hospice nurse indicated that using the belt in that manner constituted a restraint and that none of them could use a restraint. So be it! I can and will because it adds to her safety.

I was in the basement and there was a crash from above. I had left her sleeping in the recliner. I immediately knew the problem. She wanted to get out of the recliner and didn't understand how to lower it from the reclined position. She just started to crawl out over the raised foot and the chair tipped and dumped her on the floor. There she lay on the floor but was unhurt. She said she wanted to get out of the chair but no one was there. She only weighs 118 pounds which is a huge amount for an old guy like me. First, I tried to lift her with the gait belt but couldn't. Then, I started moving her up a foam rubber wedge and gained a small amount of distance off the floor. I positioned the wheel chair close and at a good angle. I then made the final lift with her firmly planting her good leg to give me some assistance. I put her in the wheel chair and attached the gait belt as a restraint. I will not leave her unattended in the recliner again without some kind of safety restraint.

We have been struggling with the sleep issue at night. It seems that every second night is a sleepless night for us both. Last night was the night for sleeplessness again. As the evening wore on, it became apparent that there would be no sleep at all for this night. I have some oxycodone that was prescribed for pain so, in desperation, she was given one tablet to see if maybe it would aid in her sleeping. It did! About one hour after giving the tablet she became sleepy and drifted off. She was able to sleep the entire night uninterrupted. It was necessary during the night to rearrange the sheets and blankets to keep her covered but she had a good and restful sleep. These events were relayed to the hospice nurse who contacted the doctor. A prescription medication was delivered to be used as needed for insomnia. The prescription indicated that one 5 mg tablet should be given at bedtime as needed for insomnia. After some consideration, I decided to cut one of the tablets in half and give it at bedtime and if needed the other half could be given a little later. The other half was not needed. She had a good and long restful sleep.

Hopefully I am getting a little smarter in the duties of a caregiver. The bathroom has always presented a significant challenge in getting her clothes lowered, getting her onto the toilet, getting the clothes back on, and getting her back into the wheel chair. I have finally found a system that works for us. I help her to a standing position in front of the wheel chair and then have her put both of her arms around my neck. We carefully move in front of the toilet and I tell her that I am going to lower her clothes. I start to lower her clothes and if she starts to resist, I have her replace her arms around my neck then finish lowering the clothes and gently lower her to the toilet seat. When she is finished, we just do the same process in reverse. It seems to work well today. Who knows what tomorrow will bring. It seems that things are constantly changing and when old ways will no longer work, we have to find new ways. That is just care giving.

I read a recent article in our local newspaper titled "Dementia Costliest U. S. Malady". The Rand Corp. did a study and concluded that 4.1 million Americans have dementia. They went on to say that it is the most costly disease to society and outpaces the costs associated with heart disease and cancer. The direct costs from medicines to nursing homes are $109 billion a year in 2010 dollars. Those totals do not include informal care costs by family members and others which would push the costs significantly higher. I guess misery loves company. Assuming that the Rand Corp. study is correct, there are over 4 million people today facing the same challenges that I am facing as a caregiver.

Yesterday, I received an email from her doctor. It was a short message and was just inquiring about how I am doing. She indicated that the hospice people are keeping her well informed about my Sweetheart. I was rather shocked to receive it but it was rather comforting to think that a doctor with such a busy schedule would show concern.

Grocery shopping was on the agenda for today. Our church ladies organization had previously furnished me with a list of names of people who said they would be available to stay with my wife when I had errands to run. I attempted to call several of them today for assistance.

No help was available so I loaded her in the car and we went grocery shopping. I guided her wheel chair with one hand and pulled a grocery cart with the other hand. It was a bag your own groceries type store and it was a little difficult bagging as there was no space for parking the wheel chair. With her bad hip, we had difficulty getting her out of the car at the store and back into the car after the shopping. In both cases a kind hearted person observed our difficulty and provided some assistance. The help was definitely needed at the time and it was sincerely appreciated.

Life is constantly changing. Problems of the past are no longer problems and in their place we find new problems. We have been married for over 55 years and during all of those years my Sweetheart has always slept on the left side of the bed. Now she is sleeping in a hospital bed but I am still sleeping on the right side. Her side of the bed is more convenient but I just haven't been able to force myself to change. She had this fixation with paper and was constantly folding napkins, toilet tissue, and paper towels neatly and stacking them up. We had folded paper everyplace. She no longer has that fixation with paper. She has closets full of clothing but now is limited on what she can wear. Buttons, snaps and zippers are just too confusing for her to cope with. I have disposed of some of her clothing but much more needs to go. I just haven't been able to make myself approach that task.

I have always been an early riser. Typically, each morning, I read the newspaper and then do something on the computer. My Sweetheart would frequently come down to the basement walking very softly and attempt to startle me as I sat at the computer. My day still starts the same. As I sit at the computer I find myself constantly looking over my shoulder to see if she has come to the basement. That is a silly thing to do because she hasn't been to the basement in months. I find myself constantly pondering some of the little things that were insignificant in our lives but are now just great memories. It is sometimes hard to realize that things will never be the same and that in the not too far distant future there will be nothing left except memories. Enjoy the moment, enjoy the day, and most of all enjoy the memories.

I awoke this morning at 4 AM and was unable to get back to sleep. I lay there pondering where we are and where we are going and came to a horrible realization. I believe we may have just entered another era of care giving responsibilities. Yesterday was a little different day. She has always been able to rise to a standing position but yesterday it seemed that could only be accomplished with great difficulty. The tasks of getting her into and out of bed, onto the commode or toilet, into the shower, into the wheel chair and into the recliner seemed almost impossible. Was it that she just physically could no longer rise to a standing position or was it that she didn't understand that she needed to? I don't have an answer but today should bring one. No longer able to stand means bedridden. Not a pleasant thought.

I was in the kitchen at 6 AM and decided this was the morning for sausage, eggs, and hash-brown potatoes. I don't indulge to that extent very often but decided that this was the morning. I was midway through the cooking and thought that I heard a sound. I automatically looked up to see if she was walking down the hallway to the kitchen as she would often do in the early morning. Then I realized that she would never <u>walk</u> down that hallway again.

My Sweetheart coined a new word/phrase today. She said "I'm a loveburger". When she first used that phrase, it made me smile. Well, she has always been a dark headed beauty. However, in her mid-teenage years, she started having grey hair appear. By the time she was in her late 20's, her hair was kind of a salt and pepper mix. Not long after that she started coloring her hair as near as possible to the natural color. She always applied the coloring herself until that was no longer possible then the task fell to me. Later on we found a lady who did hair in her home and she applied the coloring until that was no longer possible. This morning the task fell back upon me and I planned to use the "Just for Men" product because of the ease of application. Squirt it on the hair, rub it to a lather, wait 5 minutes, rinse out the color and apply shampoo. I prepared her for a shower and where she can't stand we use a shower bench. It is about 4 feet long, has four legs, and has a commode hole in one end. I place one end in the bathtub and the other end outside. She sits on the outside end, slides to the inside end with the commode hole and we shower her with a hand held shower. I mixed and applied the product and waited the five minutes. Then I proceeded to do the rinse and shampoo which went well. Finally, I needed to finish the shower—then I smelled something. There it was, a big pile of poop right under the commode hole end of the shower bench. The nurse is always concerned about bowel movements but there is no need for concern today. All in all, it really wasn't such a bad day.

Today ended up being another day in the saga of bowel movements. Some three days after the above experience, she started off the day with a small bowel movement, all in the toilet. About mid-day another which was not in the toilet. Then just about bed time another and again at midnight. It was a constant clean-up effort from bedtime until 1 AM. One was a cleanup at the toilet, one a cleanup at the bedside commode and the last was a cleanup of the hospital bed, mattress and bedding. Having had a wide range of cleanup experiences, the cleanup while lying on the bed appears to be the best way. I certainly wouldn't advise anyone to purposely test my conclusion.

We have a small TV set in our kitchen. The remote control has frequently been an issue as she would put it in unusual places where it would often take days to locate. Of late the TV remote control problem has become a non-issue and we often leave it laying on the kitchen table or a cabinet close by. Today it almost ended up being a casualty. As we were eating lunch, my Sweetheart kept trying to eat the remote control. She would repeatedly attempt to take a bite then lay it down and in just a moment attempt another bite. I could not convince her that the remote control should not be eaten. Finally it was moved so it was out of sight.

It seems that the "go to" food for now is Oatmeal/Raisin Cookies. There is lots of good stuff in those cookies and she will eat one just about any time. I ask her if she wants a cookie and if she says yes, then give her a cookie and she will eat it. When she says no, lay a cookie in front of her and in just a few minutes she will be eating that cookie. How long will this last? I haven't a clue but you can rest assured it won't last all that long and then we will need to find another "go to" food.

Last night was another one of those restless nights. When she went to bed, she immediately went to sleep but then started tossing and turning. I must have covered her at least a dozen times. At 4 AM, it appeared that the night was ended and that the only alternative was to dress her for the day. Today being shower day, dressing her for the day was not a good alternative either. Finally, I decided to just change her diaper and see what happened. After the wet diaper change, she immediately fell asleep in what appeared to be a sound and restful sleep. Maybe the tossing and turning was her attempt to give me a message but I wasn't listening.

This was a play day for me. I needed to have her ready for the day when the caregiver arrived. She was alert and later on in the day she was talking and making sense. At one time, one of our sons called on the telephone and inquired about his Mom. I handed her the telephone and she carried on a conversation for several minutes. I could naturally only hear one side of the conversation but it certainly sounded like a conversation that made sense. These kinds of days are becoming less and less frequent and I'm fearful that in a short time they will only be a memory.

We celebrated Mother's Day today with all of our family except for one granddaughter. It was a good day and possibly the best Mother's Day ever. She didn't know the name of anyone but she knew they were family and she enjoyed talking with them. One of our sons said that he had read something that indicated that dementia patients frequently enjoy holding and cuddling a small baby doll. He bought one and she thoroughly enjoys it.

I was in the process of applying some preparation H and replaced the tube in the box. I pushed open the other end of the box and her dementia ID necklace fell out. I have been looking for that necklace for months but now there is no need since she is confined to a wheel chair when we are away from home. However, one of the lost is now found.

We have been preparing for the five day respite visit. That is the five day period when my wife will be placed in a care facility and I should have five days of complete freedom. At times I had concerns about it really happening. As the time grew shorter for the visit to start, more and more information was available. Clothing and other items needed packed, clothing needed marked, paperwork needed completed, and medications needed packaged.

I prepared a Respite Care Information paper and delivered it to the care facility in advance. In that paper I outlined what I considered to be essential information that would assist them in providing care and aid in her comfort. There were 14 points of information which outlined her limitations, procedures that I used in giving her care, when and how certain aspects of care were given, and clothing that was provided. In retrospect, I don't believe that information was shared with any of the caregivers in the facility.

At the appointed time on the appointed day she was dropped off at the facility where we were met by the Hospice nurse and various personnel from the care facility. The process seemed to go well and I departed for my time away. That all sounds great but I had this nagging feeling that I was neglecting something and my thoughts were almost constantly about her welfare. I have a cell phone that is kept in our car and it is only used when I am away from my Sweetheart. The first night that I was away, I turned off the cell phone and laid it on a night stand. In the middle of the night I awoke and came to the realization that I should have the cell phone turned on in case the care facility needed to contact me. I immediately turned it on and checked for any messages.

I returned home a day early and brought her home from the care facility a day early. There was no sign at all of recognition and she seemed in a stupor for all of the day and into the evening. Two of our sons visited her regularly and there were some instances that one son noted that casts some doubt on the quality of care. Later in the day I was going through the bubble packed medications and noted that one of her medications was not given at any time during her stay. That particular medication has been taken for several years and when it is started or stopped, it must be carefully administered to gradually increase or decrease the dosage over an extended time period. In addition, when I changed the narcotic pain patch it was noted that three days earlier when the facility changed the patch that the old patch was not removed. She has been wearing two patches for three days which definitely results in over medication. It appears that the failure to give a medication and failure to remove the old pain patch when the new one was applied are pure cases of neglect on the part of the facility. Those failures coupled with other instances brings into consideration a serious question as to the quality of care. This will definitely become a major topic of consideration with the Hospice nurse at the earliest possible time. Although it is not a shortcoming of the Hospice provider, it should be of concern to them for future respite care for all of their patients.

I put things in writing. I don't like to rely on word of mouth which can result in poor communication and misinterpretation. I have fully documented the above noted experiences and issues and furnished copies to Hospice. They have assured me that the issues will be addressed with appropriate personnel in the care facility.

The respite absence was for three nights and four days. The failure to give the required medication and the overmedication with the pain patch have, in my opinion, taken a toll. It seems that she sleeps excessively and is more difficult to manage than she has been in the past. Caregiver tasks that were simple and routine last week are now difficult and demanding. I'm sure it will be several days until she recovers. Last evening she was sitting in the living room in her wheel chair when I came into the room from being outside. She recognized me and threw her arms open wide in a greeting. That is the first recognition that I have noted since her return home from the respite absence. Hopefully things are on the mend.

I had an off day yesterday and did some real relaxing. I went to lunch alone. That is the first time I have been to lunch alone in a very long time. Take it from me, it was not enjoyable at all. There was just a feeling of emptiness and loneliness during the entire time. I know that I will have to become accustomed to that feeling as things will never improve.

Things constantly change. Each morning I leave the house and walk to the roadway to pick up my newspaper. I always unlock the front door dead bolt and the locking mechanism on the door knob, walk onto the front step, check the door knob to make sure it is unlocked, and close the door. Over the years there have been a few times that I have locked myself out of the house. No problem, I could just ring the doorbell and wake my Sweetheart who could come and open the door. That is not the case any longer. I have several house keys stashed at various places in the event that I am locked out.

It is hard for me to realize that she can no longer move about the house unless she is placed in a wheel chair and moved by someone. She hasn't been to the basement in months and likely will never visit it again. We have a large yard and significant yard work is required. When she naps in the recliner I can do yard work but must constantly check to assure she is doing well. On those days when yard work is required and she doesn't nap, I place her in the wheel chair and move her outside where she can observe me working. When the day is very warm, she is positioned in sight of where I am working but in a shady area. She enjoys going outside and watching the yard work progress.

It took me sometime to realize that some assistance was needed in carrying the load. I had decided that I needed a paid person for two days each week and eight hours each day but later changed that to seven hours each day. Through our church I was given the name of a person who was interested in the paid caregiver position. After an interview with her she was offered the position but later declined. Before her declination, another person was interviewed and it seemed she was a much better fit and had better qualifications. She later accepted the position and has been a godsend in providing loving care.

Caller ID and phone mail are great improvements to telephone systems but, in my opinion, are greatly misused. Far too many people will receive a telephone call, look at the caller ID and then not answer the telephone because they don't wish to talk to the caller. Many people will never answer a telephone call in person but just use the phone mail to take a message and then decide if they want to return the call. The typical message "I'm either on the telephone or away from my desk" makes my blood boil.

I was recently given a list of several people from our church who apparently said they were willing to provide assistance for short periods of time when I needed to visit a doctor, dentist, shop for groceries or an absence for other purposes. After making at least a dozen telephone calls to those same people on days when I needed assistance and never getting any answer, I am convinced that I was victimized by caller ID and phone mail abuse. When it comes to getting assistance from other people it is my opinion that people can be divided into four categories. Category I – can't help. Category II - won't help. Category III – will help. Category IV – they stand up before their peers (to impress them) and offer to help but have no intention at all of helping if they are called. The only person you can count on is yourself so you had better figure out a way to do things yourself.

We just celebrated our wedding anniversary after 55 years of marriage. The day before our anniversary we drove to a local bulk flower outlet and purchased several bunches of flowers. We took them home to clip and arrange them as I thought my wife would enjoy doing the arranging. She was not interested at all but was content just sitting and watching. I am not a good flower arranger but we did get the job done. The day of our anniversary I needed to do a few errands and purchase some items to make our anniversary somewhat memorable. The assistance that I was planning on did not materialize. It became necessary for me to move her to the car drive a few miles and then place her in the wheel chair. We spent over an hour at that business then back into the car and drive a few more miles. Then, out of the car and into the wheel chair again but in that process she nearly fell. We spent another hour with me pushing the wheel chair with one hand and pulling a shopping cart with the other hand. As we were exiting that store we met a long-time acquaintance whose first question was "why are you doing this, can't you get some help"? Then back into the car and our next stop where my Sweetheart stayed in the car. The entire trip consumed several hours and could have been done in less than half the time had the assistance been available. Our 55th wedding anniversary was indeed a memorable day. It will not be fondly remembered because it was full of disappointments. Whose fault was that – mine. I should never have planned on any assistance from anyone. Maybe I need to discontinue doing things I <u>want</u> to do on paid caregiver days and do all of my errands, doctor appointments and shopping.

We are struggling with the bowel movement problem. It seems they are too frequent or not frequent enough. For a period of time I was giving a small daily dose of a mild laxative resulting in the BM being too frequent. I stopped the daily dose and gave a partial dose every three days which is not working. I'm now attempting to get her started again by giving her a full dose two times a day. After one day with two doses she started and had 7 BMs in a 24 hour period. Not good! I won't do that again.

Things seem to be in constant change. Just when it seems that I have everything figured out, then something changes. During one of her recent BM accidents I was trying to change her lying on the bed. In the process, her elastic waist trousers needed removed and it resulted in a terrible mess. Rather than put elastic waist trousers on her the next time, I put on an elastic waist full skirt. It seems much better and easier to work with when assisting her with bathroom issues. I'm not ready to completely discontinue the use of trousers but in the future they will not be used exclusively.

Several months ago we purchased a recliner and a flat screened TV for the living room. The thought was that when she wanted to rest and nap, just put her in the recliner. She never was really satisfied with the recliner and often complained when placing it in the reclined position. During the last few days when she wanted to rest and nap the hospital bed was used. She seems much more content lying in the hospital bed and if an accident happens or if she needs to be changed then there is no need to move her. I'm not sure how long this system will last but it works well until something better comes along.

I love fresh corn on the cob and good whole kernel corn. We have always looked forward to the time of year when the fresh corn was available at roadside stands and in farmers markets. I'm sure you are well aware that when corn passes through your system and comes out the other end, it is still recognizable. A person who wears diapers and frequently has accidents should not be fed whole kernel corn. It is not only bad for them but is also bad for the person who must change the diapers. We have this kind hearted lady who has been bringing us food periodically. She makes great soups but the problem is they are loaded with whole kernel corn. How does a person tactfully tell a kind hearted lady who out of the goodness of her heart is going to great effort to give us prepared food that the whole kernel corn is a problem? I have been pondering that issue now for some time and just haven't found the answer.

It seems there is always a problem regulating the amount of laxative to give on a daily basis. We have tried Miralax which seems to work best and we have tried various dosages. It has been necessary to stop and start at various times but have been trying to determine a standard daily dose that works. At the present time I am giving her ½ teaspoon (carefully measured) in her juice each morning. That dosage seems to be working but not sure how long that will continue.

In the past we have frequently eaten in a restaurant somewhat regularly. With the difficulty getting her into and out of a vehicle, those restaurant trips have become less and less frequent. This past evening we ventured to a restaurant again and it was a very pleasant experience. It was unbelievable how much food she consumed. She was alert and appeared to thoroughly enjoy the restaurant experience. We may have to venture out more often.

How do you occupy a person who has dementia? Mostly it is sleep, eat, sit and look at pictures or magazines and then sleep again. Most days seem to follow that routine. Part of today was a little different. She has a small writing notebook that she carefully guards. I have printed a few simple words or names on some of the pages and she will often study them carefully. I often give her a pencil in case she wants to write or draw something on the pages. Today seemed to be an intense day. She sat at the kitchen table for hours studying the notebook and scribbling on some of the pages. She also had a bath towel over her legs which she took and folded using it to wrap the notebook. It was a good day that I will remember and hopefully she will have many more.

Today is paid caregiver day and my day to play. I was putting my golf clubs in the trunk of the car this morning and in the process, the wheel chair needed removed. Also, in the bottom of the trunk is a storage compartment where we have extra coats, small blankets, small pillows and various other items. While I was storing some of the items which had been removed, the thought struck me – why? There is absolutely no need to carry those items in the car any longer but I just can't force myself to remove them. She will not be travelling any distance where those items would be needed. Then I began thinking about the can and can'ts, the dos and don'ts, and the will and won'ts. The list gets longer and longer as each day goes by. She can't walk or stand or get into bed or get out of bed or get into the wheel chair or get out of the wheel chair without help. In fact, there are very few things that she can do. She does feed herself most of the time but there are occasions when she must be fed. Although the list of can'ts, won'ts and don'ts gets longer, I look forward to doing those things for her. I know that if the tables were turned and she was the caregiver, the quality of care that I would receive far surpasses anything that I could do. When the day comes when my caregiver duties are ended just think of the great memories that I will have.

Sometimes I don't pay attention to some of the little things that I should. I have noticed that although she doesn't know me, our children, our grandchildren, or even know her own name, there are some things that she seems to remember. She has always been very particular about her clothing and her appearance. Anytime she sees a mirror she immediately starts trying to fix her hair so that every hair is in just the right place. Most of the time she doesn't make an issue out of clothing but there are times when she will say that a certain combination just doesn't look right. Today she had on a blue and white blouse and the blue skirt needed washed. I put a maroon skirt on her and she immediately said she needed another blouse because the blue one didn't match. I gave her a matching blouse and all was well.

I am an early riser. I have this internal alarm cloth that wakes me at about 5 AM. I have repeatedly tried to reset that internal clock but without success. I just get out of bed at 5 AM, go to the basement to shave, shower and dress. Then, I read my paper and watch the news until about 8 AM when she normally is awake. This morning I had an outside project and wanted to work while the temperatures were cool. I started the project at 6 AM and at 7:45 AM it was finished. I immediately came inside to check on her. Some way she had gotten the side rails removed from the bed and was laying on the floor of the bedroom busying herself by picking up lint from the carpet. We struggled to get her off the floor and into the wheel chair but were finally successful. After she was dressed I realized that I hadn't put on her slippers. I went to the bedroom to retrieve them and they were not in the normal place where they are always kept. I found them inside a plastic bag that was placed under a wardrobe along with several other items that she had neatly stored away.

Cookies, brownies, cake, pies, rolls and you name it! The caregiver who comes in two days each week is always making something. I look forward to what is coming next and my Sweetheart just likes to eat it. The hospice nurse has said that maybe we need to get more protein into her diet. I guess we probably should but why? A person with dementia has few pleasures in life and if one of them is eating sweet things then I say they should eat them. I haven't a clue on what the life expectancy will be but they should eat what they enjoy and if their life is shortened by some small amount of time, then so be it.

I was thinking about the "Forest Gump" movie and the saying that "Life is like a box of chocolates". Care giving is very similar because we never know what the next day will bring. Things may be going very smoothly and all of a sudden, for no apparent reason, they change drastically. I normally give her a shower and shampoo every Sunday and the only resistance is when it comes to the shampoo. That has been the case since I first started providing shower assistance. This last Sunday there was resistance from the time she entered the shower. I'm always looking for ways to change things to make care giving more workable. Sometimes it is the little things and sometimes major changes are needed. Breakfast is usually cereal of some kind but we change that periodically. Just yesterday, breakfast was cereal which was sprinkled generously with raisins. She has never been a big raisin fan but yesterday she thoroughly enjoyed them. Her eating habits are changing and she is eating less and less with utensils. A person could make an issue of her eating habits but what difference does it make? The important thing is that she is eating and seems to be enjoying it. It is certainly less stressful on both parties to just accept that she will be eating more with her fingers.

Every day is a good day, some better than others but all are good days and leave us with memories. I am sure that as time goes by we will cling to those memories and vividly recall some of the good times. We have positioned her hospital bed at the foot of the master bed. Tonight she was laying in the hospital bed trying to sleep but was very restless. I moved down to the foot of the master bed and took her hand so she would know that I was near. She gently kissed my hand and whispered "I love you" as she drifted into a deep sleep.

And thus ended the third day.

CHAPTER 4

The Fourth Day

And God said, Let there be lights in the firmament of the heaven to divide the day from the night; and let them be for signs and for seasons, and for days, and for years: And let them be for lights in the firmament of the heaven to give light upon the earth: and it was so. And God made two great lights; the greater light to rule the day, and the lesser light to rule the night: he made the stars also. And God set them in the firmament of the heaven to give light upon the earth, And to rule over the day and over the night, and to divide the light from the darkness: and God saw that it was good. Genesis 1:14-18

The Hospice Nurse visits two times each week. She takes vital signs, checks for bed sores and offers suggestions on how to better care for my Sweetheart. During her most recent visit, she indicated that maybe more effort should be made to increase the protein in her diet. My wife lost her sense of taste years ago but can detect sweet and sour tastes. As a general rule, she loves sweet foods. Her quality of life leaves much to be desired and there are few things that give her pleasure. I am of the opinion that if she enjoys sweet foods then she should have every opportunity to enjoy them. If that means she has a poor diet then so be it. Let her enjoy to the fullest one of the few pleasures of her life.

Alfred Dunner slacks are a godsend. They are the polyester slacks with no buttons, snaps or zippers and have an elastic waist. I bought her about half a dozen pair and was very particular to get the correct size. They looked nice, were easy to put on and take off, and washed very well. They worked great until she started wearing diapers twenty four hours a day. Now it is a struggle to put them on and take them off because of the added bulk generated by the diapers. We started with a size 8P then one of our sons bought her two pair of size 10P. They didn't go on or off any easier. I just visited the local J C Penny's store and purchase two more pair – size 14P. They still look good and are much easier to manage. Finally though we settled on size 18P as being the best size and in the capri style then the length doesn't need to be altered.

Along with all of the other issues to contend with, we were informed today that she has shingles. She had a shingles shot so hopefully they won't be quite so severe. The pharmacy delivered the medication and she must take 1 tablet 3 times each day for seven days. The tablets are huge and contain 1,000 mg. The first dose was crushed and put in a drink but would not completely dissolve so the residue was given in a spoonful of strawberry jam. The next dose was crushed, sprinkled on buttered toast with honey and cinnamon. That method worked well. By experimenting it was found that crushing and mixing with liquid will work well but it must sit in the liquid for about 30 minutes before it is completely dissolved. Some kind of sweetener needs adding because of the very bitter taste.

Her prescription medications are ordered from the doctor by Hospice and the pharmacy delivers them to our home. The shingles medication was delivered on a Friday. The following Monday, another delivery of shingles medication was made but was only for 5 days. Before accepting I contacted the Hospice nurse and inquired as to why another delivery. She told me that apparently the doctor had determined that she should take the medication for 12 days rather than the original 7 days. I noted that two different doctors had ordered the medications. I sent her regular doctor an email and asked for clarification as to how long my wife should take the medication, 7 days or 5 days or 12 days. Her regular doctor responded that she should take the medication for 7 days and that the 5 day prescription from another doctor was written by a PA (Physician Assistant) working in pediatrics in a completely different office. The following day, the pharmacy attempted to deliver yet another prescription for shingles medication from the pediatric PA.

I recently returned home after a few days away. The hired caregiver had agreed to stay in our home and provide care in my absence. Shortly after my departure a new prescription was delivered by the pharmacy. Upon my return, I noted the new prescription which was some kind of powerful pain medication and started to do some research. I then came to the realization that the prescription was not for my wife but had been delivered to the wrong address. This instance is the second problem with medications which were delivered by this pharmacy.

It seems that each day she loses some of her skills. The changes are very gradual but as one looks back they are easily recognizable. Her eating habits are making more use of her fingers and less use of utensils. I find myself feeding her a great deal of the time depending upon the type of food she is eating. Seldom will she tell you if she is hungry or thirsty but if you ask, she will often give a response. She takes her medications really quite well. At times she does not swallow them and later a part of a pill can be found where she has put it. When that happens, I crush the remaining part of the pill and put it in a spoonful of jam or jelly. She normally has one or two bowel movements each day but they are hardly ever in the toilet. When she is put on the toilet she will usually urinate. She seldom is willing to do the paperwork after using the toilet. Hospice furnishes a spray that is very effective in cleaning her after a bowel movement. I usually lay her on a towel on the hospital bed to do the clean-up.

I decided that her new trousers needed to be shortened. That didn't appear to be a big problem, just take the scissors and cut some off. I did and then put them in the washing machine. When I removed them, the bottom of the legs were terribly frayed. No problem, they just need to be hemmed. I don't know how to operate the sewing machine and could not find an instruction booklet. I finally gave up and called a neighbor for some help but she isn't a seamstress. I found a needle and thread and decided I would try and hem them by hand. The problem was the eye of the needle was so small that I couldn't see to thread it. I tried threading it looking through a magnifying glass but that didn't help. I finally found a needle with a large enough eye and started the hemming process. The job was completed in about an hour and didn't look that bad to me but would probably give a real seamstress nightmares. I'm not sure that I want to shorten anymore of her trousers but I did get the job done.

There are times after visiting the bathroom that fully dressing her again is not practical. At those times, she is put back into the wheel chair wearing a blouse or sweater on top and the diaper on the bottom. I would always find something to cover her such as a light blanket or large towel. We have several barbeque aprons which are used frequently for a bib when she is eating. They work very effectively for that and will cover the front and lower extremities. I also determined that they would be a great benefit to use as a cover when she is in the wheel chair with no trousers or skirt or diaper. I may have to shop for more of those aprons for future use.

I awoke at about 11 PM to this terrible smell. I asked if she had pooped in her pants and the response that I got was "probably". Usually there is no response or one which doesn't make sense. I changed her and hoped she would go back to sleep immediately. Not so! She tossed & turned, muttered, sang and hummed most of the night away. Finally about 5 AM she drifted off to sleep. Today is normally a shower day but that and her breakfast may be delayed because of her sleeplessness.

I have come to the realization that the closets and drawers full of clothing and shoes are no longer needed. In fact, except for a few items, none of the clothing or shoes will ever be worn again. I hesitate to take them to a local charitable organization because of the quality and my sentimental attachment but also realize that they are of no use. My first thought was to offer them to family members which I am in the process of doing. I'm sure that some of the items will be well received and appreciated.

Today was a good day. There was no nap but the entire day was spent visiting, arranging personal items and looking at photo albums. She has two empty golf ball boxes, one pink and one blue. She has them filled with her own personal treasures. She is constantly removing the items from the boxes, moving to the other box or just looking them over and replacing them in the boxes. She seems to get a great deal of pleasure from doing those things. During the process today, I came to the realization that she needs a small table in the living room where she can sit in her wheel chair and have a work area. We have a card table that should work well. Sometimes it is the small and insignificant things that makes life just a little better.

Yes, the card table worked well in the living room. I moved her wheel chair up to the card table and placed two photo albums there for her. I also found another empty golf ball box to put on the table with some small items inside. She spent several hours completely engrossed in looking at albums and rearranging the personal items in the small box. One of the items in the box was a small porcelain song bird. She tried several times to eat it so it was removed and put out of sight. She seemed to thoroughly enjoy using the table and it will become a permanent fixture in the future.

Her night medication consists of two small pills. She usually puts them into her mouth with no problems and then she is given water to drink and assist her in swallowing the pills. As she is drinking, I always tell her to swallow the pills. About a half hour after her pills were given she held something up and said "come and take this". It was one of her night pills which was partially dissolved. I took the pill, crushed it, and mixed it with a teaspoon full of jam which she readily ate. The thought immediately crossed my mind as to how many times she has done this same thing without my knowledge. Tonight when I gave her the night medications, I used the same procedure but after the water, I gave her several pieces of caramel popcorn which she loves. She immediately chewed and swallowed it which assures that the pills were also swallowed. I may want to keep a supply of caramel popcorn or some other small treat on hand to help her swallow the medications.

A lady from our church had called and asked if she could bring some young people to our home to play some music for my Sweetheart. They were scheduled to arrive at 7 PM. She also asked her favorite dessert so we could have some refreshments after the music. A short time before their arrival, we placed a note on the door that we were in the back yard and to come back and join us. We then retired to our private forest in our backyard and started a small campfire. When they arrived we were sitting by the fire in the late evening enjoying the outdoors. We were then treated to an outstanding program by three young people, ages 11, 12 and 15, playing their stringed instruments. After the musical program we were then served ice cream and brownies. My wife was served first. After she had finished her dessert, she looked over at me and noticed that I was still eating my dessert. She said "I want that", pointing to my ice cream and brownie. I traded dishes with her and she happily finished my dessert. It was indeed a great day.

Our middle son and one of his daughters came to visit this past weekend. We were playing in a two man golf tourney and the grand daughter who is a CNA was planning on caring for my wife while my son and I were on the golf course. I had some reservations about our granddaughter's ability to provide the necessary care but those concerns were soon banished when we were preparing her for bed. It became readily apparent to me that she had the knowledge and the skills to provide the care far better than I. When we came back home after the first day of play, my wife was sporting nail polish on both hands. When I asked our granddaughter how it was possible for her to apply the nail polish she told me that she just removed everything from her table and was able to apply the polish with no problems. We had a very enjoyable visit and our oldest son with his wife and our youngest son spent considerable time visiting. My Sweetheart did not know the name of anyone but during the course of one of the visits she exclaimed "this is my family". That was another example of what I believe to be the small flashes of clarity that people with dementia have from time to time.

A short time ago the hospice nurse asked how she was doing with her teeth brushing. I informed her that she hadn't brushed her teeth in months. Although significant efforts were made, she just refused to brush. I had tried assisting, encouraging and brushing for her but all attempts had failed. The nurse suggested that maybe I should give her some chewing gum. I expressed my concern that she would swallow it but the nurse assured me that it would not be a health problem if she did. I secured some gum and have been giving it to her several times each day for over a week. In all that time she has swallowed the gum only one time. She is reluctant to remove it from her mouth when asked but I have found that if I offer her some caramel popcorn that she will readily remove the gum. It seems I am finding more and more benefits to having caramel corn readily available.

Quite frequently she will be in need of a nap during the day. In those instances she is usually placed on the hospital bed and covered with a sheet. She seems to rest much better than in the recliner. She was sitting at her table rearranging her treasures and had yawned several times. I asked if she was tired and wanted to take a short nap. Her response was "no I don't want to take a nap, I'm just stretching my mouth."

About 10 months ago she started losing weight. Her appetite at that time was terrible and I was trying various ways to encourage her to eat. She continued to lose weight and in a four month period she had lost over 40 pounds. Since that time her appetite has improved and she has gained back about 20 pounds. She has an excellent appetite but I will need to monitor her weight closely in the future.

I am constantly amazed at the response she gives to questions. Mostly when she is asked something, she will give a response that makes absolutely no sense at all. But there are times when her response makes complete sense and is even shocking. A real advantage to caring for someone with dementia is that when they get upset or mad, it is usually forgotten in just a few seconds. She was recently irritated at something that I had done and in fact was quite upset. I waited a few seconds and asked her if she knew who I was and did she love me. Her response was "sometimes."

In the past when I have written in my "Diary of a Caregiver", I have positioned myself at the computer and written. Now, I have at hand a notepad where I can capture on paper those rare moments that I believe warrant recording. A few moments ago we were sitting at the breakfast table waiting for shower time. I told my Sweetheart "You just look beautiful this morning." Her response was a wide grin, a gesture with her arms and a slight nod of her head as if to simulate a bow. She doesn't know me, she doesn't know our grown children or our grandchildren but she still has her sense of humor. In my opinion, a sense of humor is so important not only for the Caregiver but also for the Patient.

Looking back in time just one year ago and how things were then as compared to now, a person can recognize that significant changes have occurred. No longer can she read anything, not even her own first name. When you ask her to do something, she doesn't understand. When you ask her a question, she doesn't give you an answer. The list goes on and seems to be without end. There are times though when she seems quite normal and responds to questions but those times are few and far between. She still has a good sense of humor and is really quite pleasant at most times. She spends large amounts of time at her table with her things arranging and rearranging.

She has been eating well for some time now and has gained back about 20 pounds of the 40 she had lost. One never knows what she will enjoy eating but seems to dislike most kinds of meats. She will always eat toast smothered with jam or jelly but it must be served open faced and cut into small pieces that she can eat with a fork. I often give her various kinds of fruits also cut into small pieces. One morning when I was very shaky while attempting to slice up a banana, I remarked to her about my shakiness and she responded with "just cut off a hunk and give it to me." I did and she ate it even though she sometimes refuses to eat bananas. She seems to always enjoy oatmeal cookies and also brownies. With her recent weight gain there is concern that she may continue to gain which could be a problem. I am in the process of changing her drinks so they will be lower in calories and assist in stabilizing her weight. The latest weight shows that she gained 2 pounds in two weeks.

This was a weepy day! That is a day when it seems that she just sits and cries for no apparent reason. When you ask her why she is crying, her response is that she doesn't know and then she keeps crying. At bedtime tonight it was especially bad. She cried when I removed her slippers. She cried when I removed her trousers. She cried when I removed her diaper. She cried when I sat her on the commode. She cried while she sat on the commode. She cried when I put on the new and clean diaper. She cried when I sat her on the hospital bed. She cried when I laid her down and covered her with a sheet. Then, all became quiet and she seemed to be asleep immediately. Hopefully she will relax and have a restful night and awake in the morning fully rested. The nurse believes she has a urinary tract infection (UTI) and has secured a doctors order for testing. A UTI could be the cause for at least some of the crying. We will be involved in trying to get a good urine specimen for laboratory testing tomorrow.

My hopes did not materialize. She was wide awake at 11 PM and did not sleep until about 3 AM. She was running a fever of 100.9. The nurse has told me when she is running a fever to give Tylenol. The liquid is very thick and hard to measure, in addition it is difficult to get someone to drink the liquid when they can't understand your instructions. A short time ago I had washed and saved a soft drink plastic bottle. I crushed 1000 mg of Tylenol tablets, put them in the plastic bottle and then filled it partially with a bright red colored punch. I was able to raise the hospital bed and give her the bottle. She removed the cap and drank about half of the liquid containing the Tylenol. About an hour later she was able to sleep. I may have to keep several of the empty bottle for a similar future use. For some reason she drinks better from a bottle that she can hold rather than from a glass with or without a straw.

The pharmacy delivered the medication for treatment of the UTI and of course, it is 500 mg tablets and she must take one tablet per day for 7 days. She just doesn't do well with those large tablets so they must be crushed. I crushed the tablet for the first day and added about 1 cup of a sweet juice. The drink was so bitter that no one could drink it. I added artificial sweetener to no avail and finally just sat that container aside for a later date. Another tablet was crushed and mixed with strawberry jam and it was successfully given. On day number two, a pancake was cut in half, the crushed pill was sprinkled over the pancake and then smothered in strawberry jam. It was an effort but I was successful in getting her to eat it. On day three and after, I crushed the pill, put a small amount of jam in two teaspoons, added ½ of the crushed pill in each teaspoon and then topped it with more jam. That system seems to work the best. Now I am on the last day and must give her the last tablet that has been mixed with juice. I have added various juices and sweeteners to make it somewhat drinkable. What started out as one cup of juice is now over one quart but I will be successful in getting the last pill taken. Although it is quite frustrating at times, it is also challenging and when the job is done there is considerable personal satisfaction from figuring out ways to solve the problems of care giving. I know all of the problems will never be solved but that keeps life interesting and just think of all of the memories.

The morning medications are usually taken with no problems but the evening medications have become an issue. For some reason she just refuses to take the medications and pleading doesn't seem to help. A pill crusher has become a necessity and is used at least one time each day. The crushed tablets or capsule contents must be mixed with a liquid or food item and you must have some kind of assurance that the patient will be willing to consume the mixture. It seems that all of the medications have a disagreeable and bitter taste. As of now, the crushed contents are mixed with a jam or jelly which seems to mask the unpleasant taste and make the mixture appetizing to the patient.

During my entire adult life I have been concerned with my weight. I have closely monitored to assure that my weight was not excessive. At the time of my retirement some 18 years ago my weight was 195 and it was my intention to reduce my weight to 180. That was accomplished gradually over a period of years. About 2 years ago it was decided that I would reduce my weight to 170 and maintain at that level. I began drinking diet drinks and it was easy to maintain at my desired level. Now, all of a sudden, I have started losing weight again which is not of my choosing. I have discontinued drinking diet drinks and now routinely drink those with higher calories. As of this writing, my weight has dropped to 163 pounds. I need to pay more attention to my diet and increase my weight back to 170 pounds and maintain it at that level. This issue has not been brought to my primary care physician but will be should I be unsuccessful in gaining and maintaining my weight at the desired level.

We had visitors at our home last evening from our church. They came just before bedtime to visit and inquired as to our wellbeing. It was an enjoyable time and my Sweetheart was very alert and in good spirits. She would ramble on not making much sense but enjoying the company. As their visit came to a close, they suggested that they offer a prayer prior to their departure. I told my Sweetheart that they were going to offer a prayer and that she needed to fold her arms and bow her head. She needed no further urging and I am convinced that at that moment she clearly understood what was happening and why it was happening. That evening became a very memorable moment that will be cherished.

There is a website available through her primary care physician where one can look at medical records, test results, send messages to the doctor and various other items associated with her care. I was looking at some of the information and was reviewing her medications. She has recently had a medication prescribed which is a low dose antibiotic for treatment of urinary tract infection. That medication was delivered by the pharmacy about one week ago and had the instructions that it should be taken one time each day and with food or milk. The information that her doctor had entered into her medical records was "take one capsule (50 mg total) by mouth nightly." Some medications need to be taken in the morning, some at night, and some at mid-day. Unless they are taken at the proper time and in the proper dosage their effectiveness comes into question. In this particular instance, the pharmacy apparently changed the instructions given by the doctor and that is not their prerogative. This subject will be addressed further sometime in the future.

Today was shower day and the CNA needed to readjust her schedule. She arrived at 9 AM and it is usually about 10:30 AM. I gave the medications at the regular time which is about 8:30 AM and apparently that did not allow sufficient time for them to take effect before the shower. She was very uncooperative and resisted everything that needed to be done. After some time the shower was completed and within a couple of minutes after she was dressed she had forgotten that it was so unpleasant. If there is a plus side to dementia, it would have to be that unpleasant things are quickly forgotten. She has a sweet disposition and immediately reverts back to being cheerful and pleasant. There may be some bad times but really, all days are good days!

My sweetheart hasn't been for a car ride for several weeks. My sister suggested that she would enjoy being away from home and going for a long ride. I painted the following scenario for her. I would need to take some diapers in case she had an accident. There most likely would not be any adult changing stations so it would be necessary to lay her on the ground for changing. That presents the problem of getting her off the ground and into the car or wheelchair after changing. I have been instructed by Hospice that when she is on the floor or on the ground and assistance is needed that 911 should be called. They most likely would respond with an ambulance or fire engine with sirens blaring. They would provide the assistance needed to get her into the car so we could return home. Under the circumstances, going for a long car ride is not a wise choice.

Breakfast this morning was French Toast. I have often wondered why it is called "French" toast. Most likely for the same reason they have "French" fried potatoes. I prepared two pieces on two separate plates, one smothered with maple syrup and one smothered with frozen strawberry jam. I placed both plates directly in front of her at the same time. The first bite was frozen strawberry jam. I believe she was attracted by the bright color. The second bite was the maple syrup. She continued eating the maple syrup French toast until it was gone. She stopped eating for several minutes and then ate every bite of the strawberry jam French toast. I wonder if the results would be the same if a different kind of jam was used on the French toast.

It was one of those days today where she seemed to forget how to eat by herself. I would give her a bite of food and she would immediately want another but couldn't seem to understand what to do. Her food was in a dish and the only utensil needed was a spoon. She was also given a slice of toast cut in half. It became necessary to give her a bite of food and then a bite of toast. She readily ate when assisted but just refused to try to eat by herself. Our next meal she seemed to fully understand how to feed herself and ate the complete meal without any assistance.

Today was my day to play and I played. Along towards evening things started to deteriorate. It all started with me giving her the evening medications. Bad mistake on my part because rather than give her plain water to assist in the swallowing of the pills, I gave her a red colored punch. Between her not wanting to take a drink and my shakiness, the entire contents of the glass of red colored punch was spilled on the light beige carpet. I immediately began attempting to remove the stain. I tried plain water and then a high quality carpet cleaner but neither worked that successfully. In the process, I had removed a roll of paper towels from the towel holder and while replacing the roll in the holder, the end of the holder fell off. It was one of those fancy oak holders that matched our cupboards and the glue had just failed. No problem, I just needed to remove the towel holder, re-glue and reinforce with screws and then reinstall. Problem - I couldn't remove the towel holder without removing the built in microwave. I decided to attempt to reattach the end with screws working under a cupboard attached to the wall. Between my shakiness and not being able to see where I was working, the simple project turned into a major effort. I got lucky and managed to get one screw in place and attached and the rest was easy. Some of the stain still remains and I will try again tomorrow. Maybe a slight stain will be a good reminder to not do dumb things in the future.

This was the evening for resistance. She was alert and very cooperative all during the day. She took her medications without any problems and was just very pleasant. Then, bed time arrived and she seemed to resist everything that needed to be done. When I took her out of the wheel chair and sat her on the side of the hospital bed, she hung onto the hand rails of the wheel chair. It took several attempts before she could be moved. She resisted when her trousers were removed. She resisted when her diaper was removed and she was sat on the bedside commode. She resisted when we put on a clean new diaper and when she was moved back to the side of the bed. She resisted when she was laid on the bed and covered with a sheet and blanket. Then she shut her eyes and was asleep immediately.

Today I was reviewing some of the things which have happened in the past. When people inquire as to how things are going, my response is almost always "it's a good day". Granted some days are better than other days but, all days are good days. My sweetheart was put on Hospice on March 6, 2013. The following is a daily record of how things were beginning on that day and for various days for the remainder of the month. This document bears reviewing because of the turmoil in our lives at that time.

3/6 Wed – Today was doctor day for Dr. P. She put her on hospice. We had a hospice nurse and social worker visit and filled out papers. I gave her the regular meds and also gave her 2 extra Tramadols at 4 AM.

3/7 Thurs – She slept until about nine this morning. She took meds but I didn't give her a shower. The Nurse's aide came about 2 and tried to give her a shower but couldn't, tried to do her fingernail and toe nails but couldn't. She will be coming back on Monday and Thursdays. I think they are going to have to give her a pill of some kind to make her more cooperative. I had a serious problem on getting her to take her noon meds but finally got it done. We went grocery shopping with the wheel chair today. Didn't work very well. Makes it too hard to push the wheel chair and carry a basket full of groceries at the same time. Won't do that again. She hasn't eaten hardly anything today only drank some pineapple/orange juice with fresh whipped up strawberries in it. She seems to like that. She woke up at 4 AM and I gave her two tramadols. She had a total of 8 tramadols for the day.

3/8 Fri – She slept until about 10 AM this morning. I tried to wake her earlier. It took about 4 tries to get her to take her morning pills and she wouldn't shower. I noticed this morning and again this afternoon when she was napping that her hands, legs and head seem to be jerking almost constantly. She ate a good lunch – part of a pancake, some cake, and drank some lemonade spiked with blended fresh strawberries. She ate very little at dinner – just a few bites of strawberry shortcake and wouldn't drink anything. No PJs at night. Went to sleep about 9 PM and was up and down most of the night. I gave her one tramadol at 4 AM and she never went to bed after that.

3/9 Sat – She was up moving around at about 6 AM. She never slept after about 2 AM. She didn't want any food this morning but drank some juice with strawberries in. She laid down and went to sleep about 8 and I have not given her the meds yet for this morning. I gave her the meds about 10 AM – no problems – she showered but it took about 20 minutes of coaxing. She weighed 127 pounds on our scales which is down 2 pounds from 3/4. Her ear temperature was 97.8 this morning. She seemed fairly alert. She ate a small lunch and just a few bites for dinner. I only gave her 1 tramadol around 2 PM and will give her 2 more with regular meds around 7:30 PM. She refuses to remove her clothing and put on PJs. She slept pretty well but I did give her another tramadol about 4 AM. She was up at 6:30 but laid back down and went to sleep.

3/11 Mon – She was up at 7 AM. Gave her meds and she ate part of a small dish of cereal and a few bites of a sweet roll. She wouldn't drink any juice. She seems in good spirits today and we will have the Hospice CNA coming today. I have a Dr. appointment this morning. The aide arrived about 11 AM and I asked if she wanted me to stay inside or would it be best for me to leave. She said it may be better if I was to leave. A while later I came back inside and she was unable to get Marla to cooperate on having a shower. I couldn't coax her to shower either. She will be back on Thursday. I will try to get her to shower tomorrow. I noticed when I came back from the Dr. appointment that she was sitting in the chair napping and her hands and feet were shaking and jerking some. She ate a fair lunch and a fair dinner. I gave her 2 more tramadols at about 12:30 and then the evening pills at 7 PM. She doesn't want to put on PJs. A little after midnight she said her hip was hurting. I gave her 2 tramadols. At about 1 AM she said she needed to visit the bathroom. She took off her trousers and was going to put on PJs but didn't.

3/12 Tues – She was up about 8:30, took meds, showered and shampooed. It wasn't easy. She ate a very small amount of cereal for breakfast, a good lunch and very little dinner. I gave her the regular meds. We got the new med and I gave her one pill at 7 PM after several attempts. I tried to put her into PJs about 8 PM and didn't see much if any improvement in her cooperation. I may have to try two pills next time. She napped some this afternoon and was really shaky and jerky during the nap. She seems tired now and wants to go to sleep in her clothes. She became very confused and incoherent. I couldn't get her to do anything for me. During the night she spent most of it sitting on the side of the bed. I would try to get her to lay down and try to get her to visit the bathroom and mostly without success. She would sit on the side of the bed and then just lay back with her feet dangling. I would cover her and then try to sleep. At 4 AM she said she needed to visit the bathroom. She had wet the bed (the first time ever). I took her to the bathroom, she urinated, we changed her underwear and took off her trousers. I changed the bed and put it in the washer along with her wet clothes. I do not plan to give her any lorazapam at night in the future.

3/14 Thurs – Another off day for me. The aide came this morning but couldn't get her into the shower. I gave her the morning meds. She drank a little but no food for breakfast. During the day she ate well for the caregiver. The nurse came this afternoon and a new med is in the mill. She will be coming on Tuesday and Fridays. She seemed alert today and cooperated on getting her vital signs. I gave her the night meds and was able to get her into her PJ tops but failed on the bottoms. Tomorrow is shower day. She was up and down during the night. I gave her two extra tramadols at 4 AM.

3/15 Fri – I woke her up at about 9 AM. She didn't want to take her meds so am waiting until a little later. She had removed the exelon patch that I had put on her yesterday. I was able to get her into the tops of her PJs last night. This morning when she was using the toilet, I slipped off her trousers even though she resisted some but it was easy to get the PJ tops off. She wouldn't take off her underwear and started to get into the shower with them on but then removed the bottoms. She wouldn't remove the tops so I just started spraying her with the tops on. When they got wet, she removed them and went ahead and showered. She resisted the drying and dressing but we got the shower taken. She seemed somewhat disoriented this morning throughout the whole operation. I took her to get her hair colored and cut today but she wouldn't let the lady do anything. We had to just give up. She put the tops of her PJs on tonight but no bottoms. She slept very well for the entire night.

3/16 Sat – I had a hard time waking her this morning. Finally about 10 AM, I did get her up and get her to take some of her meds. I didn't give her any of the non- prescription meds for this morning. I cut back on her pain meds from 2 pills 4 X day to 1 pill 4 X day. It seemed as the day wore on that she was more alert and didn't complain any more of pain from her hip. We will see how that goes. She did have a BM today. She ate a very good lunch and a small dinner but no breakfast. She did not nap much during the day and was up and down part of the night. Maybe I have her overmedicated for pain so we will see how things go with the cutback in pain meds. She did not sleep that well and was up and down most of the night.

3/17 Sun – She was up about 8:30 this morning. I gave her the meds but only 1 tramadol this morning. I gave her another at 11 AM and then another at 2 PM. She seems to be doing well. She is alert and ate a fair lunch. Her weight this morning was 126 with clothing which is about 123 compared with previous weights. Her prior weight on 4 March – stripped was 129, a loss of 6 pounds in two weeks. She has been napping some this afternoon. She slept well tonight and she only had 4 tramadols during the day.

3/18 Mon – She was up around 9:30 and I gave her the monthly Actonel. The Aide came today and gave her a shower and shampooed her hair. She was very cooperative this morning. She had a BM this morning. She was mostly alert and quite cooperative. She ate a fair lunch and small dinner. I gave her a tramadol at midnight which makes 5 for the day. She did not sleep well during the night. She was not up roaming but seemed to be awake whenever I checked her. She put on her PJs tonight. I gave her a tramadol at midnight.

3/19 Tues – She was out of bed at 6:30 this morning. I gave her the meds. She was alert but wouldn't eat any breakfast. She just drank a small amount of juice with strawberries. She had a BM this morning. She seems a little hyper today and wouldn't take a nap. She ate a fair lunch and small dinner. She had a BM today. I gave her a total of 4 tramadols today. She put on her PJs for the night and seemed to sleep reasonably well. No up or wandering around during the night that I'm aware of. A new prescription was delivered about 8 PM, Clonazepam, but didn't have any info paper with it. I didn't give her any of the new med.

3/20 Wed – My day off. I won't give her any of the new med this morning. Maybe later in the day. I plan to look at respite facilities sometime today. The nurse called this morning and said to give the new med only when and if needed. She said if the Aide has difficulty with the shower, then give her a pill. She ate a small breakfast and seemed in good spirits while I was gone. Didn't get many answers on respite facilities. She didn't rest any during the day and at night she didn't seem to sleep at all. I gave her an extra tramadol at midnight. She ate small breakfast, a good lunch and just a few bites for dinner. I was able to get her into PJs.

3/21 Thurs – At 6 AM this morning, she was still not sleeping. I gave her one Clonazepam to see if that would quiet her down enough so she would sleep. The Aide comes today for shower and the Nurse should come at 4 PM today. I'm checking more on respite facilities today. She went to sleep and slept soundly waking at 11 AM and was given meds, dressed and went back to sleep. She was not able to get a shower this morning because she was sleeping too soundly. She was awake again at 12 noon. She ate a small lunch and a very small amount for dinner. Got her into her PJs but she didn't sleep much. At about 10:30 PM I gave her ½ of a Clonazepam. That really didn't seem to help at all. At 3:30 AM, I gave her another ½ of a Clonazepam. That didn't seem to help either. She never did really get much sleep.

3/23 Sat – Today is hair day again. I gave her the meds and the hair day turned into a disaster. The color was put on her hair without any significant problems. When it came time to shampoo, the problems started. I gave her ½ of a Clonazepam part way through the shampoo and things just got worse. She was confused and irritated and finally we had to give up. We did get her hair colored and somewhat dry but not cut. I won't give her any more clonazepam during the day. She did eat a fair breakfast and a good lunch. She had a BM today. She ate a good dinner and slept well during the night.

3/24 Sun – She woke at about 9:30 and would not shower. Gave her meds. She wouldn't eat any breakfast but ate a good lunch and dinner. She had a total of 5 tramadols today. She was quite alert. She had a BM today. I gave her a Clonazepam tonight in prep for the shower in the morning. It was 4 AM and still no sleep. She was up and down all night.

3/25 Mon – She was awake at about 9 AM and probably only slept at best 2 hours. She sat in a chair and napped the morning away. She would not eat or drink anything. The Aide came at about 11:30 but couldn't get her into the shower. She sponged her feet and legs but couldn't do anything more. I gave her another tramadol at 12:30 along with a Clonazepam. We will see what effect it has on her. Maybe I can get her into the shower a little later today. She ate a small lunch and drank 2 glasses of juice spiked with strawberries. She has great difficulty walking today with the bad hip. I have moved her around in the wheel chair most of the day. It is now 5 hours since I gave her the Clonazepam and she is still sleepy, confused and just nonfunctional. We did get her to the bathroom with great difficulty. She is better off being uncooperative at times without the Clonazepam than nonfunctional with it, in my opinion. She didn't seem to sleep much during the night. She spent most of the night sitting on the side of the bed. I would get up, put her in bed and cover her – it wouldn't be long until she was up sitting on the side of the bed again. At 5:30 AM, I tried to get her to use the bathroom but she wouldn't. I about had to carry her. I put her back into bed and at 6:30 AM she was still in bed and covered. I think I need a 4 wheeled walker with seat, it may be time for a hospital bed, and I need a ramp to wheel her out of the house to the car.

3/26 Tues – She is awake, I think, sitting on the side of the bed. She won't do anything. I tried to get her to take her meds, she wouldn't. I took the over the counter meds out and she still wouldn't take them, I crushed them and put them in a small amount of water but she wouldn't drink. I crushed them and put them in strawberry mix and she finally took them. When I try to take her to the bathroom, she won't move. As of now she will do nothing but sit. A new med was delivered today, Clonidine .1 mg. The nurse came and said to try it. I told her I probably wouldn't try it until Friday. They delivered a bedside commode but she hasn't used it yet. She took evening meds OK, no BM so I gave her a dose of Miralax. Along towards evening, she was hyper so I gave her a Clonidine .1 mg. She quieted down and slept really quite well. She sat up on the side of the bed at times but laid back down. She wouldn't get up for bathroom or to use the bedside commode.

3/27 Wed – My day off, she slept until about 11 AM gave meds and she slept some more. She was up around 2 PM and was alert. She ate a small amount for lunch and also dinner. I gave her the regular meds at about 6:30 but only gave her ½ of a Clonidine. By about 9 PM, she was getting restless and a little hyper so I gave her the other half. She had a BM today – she used the bedside commode during the night. She couldn't walk well and we wheeled her around the house. I stopped at Norco around noon and they didn't have anything processed for the 4 wheeled walker with seat. They said they would deliver it but haven't today. She is up and down tonight. We had some visitors around 5-6:30 and she got quite excited. I don't know if that contributed to her being restless and not wanting to sleep. She didn't get to sleep until around 2 AM and then has slept well.

3/28 Thurs – She was up around 8:30 and took pills. She was alert and didn't sleep much today. She ate a small amount. No BM noted. They delivered a 4 wheeled walker with seat. Have had difficulty in getting her to take night meds. She changed underwear bottoms and PJs but did not really get dressed today. She went to sleep around 9 PM and seemed to sleep good all night.

3/29 Fri – She was up about 9 AM and I had difficulty getting her to take her meds. I asked if she would like to shower and she said yes. I got her into the shower and she said the stool was cold so I covered it with a towel. She showered and we shampooed her hair. She ate no breakfast, a small lunch and a small dinner. We got a urine sample and the lab called telling us that she had a urinary tract infection. Meds were delivered about 8 PM. It appears she is going to be up most of the night. Up all night – no sleep at all.

3/30 Sat – She ate no breakfast, a fair lunch and dinner. No problems taking meds. She did not sleep any during the day. It appears that tonight may be another sleepless night. Fooled again. It took a while to get her into bed but she did sleep reasonably well. I had to put her back into bed one time during the night. No BM's noted during the day.

3/31 Sun – Will give her a dose of Miralax today. She had a BM today. Slept well and was up around 9 AM. I gave her the meds but had problems getting her to dress. We went to lunch and she ate well. She went to sleep around 9 PM and slept well – getting up twice to use bedside but went right back to sleep.

Every day seems to be interesting and one never knows what will come next. Some days she will lay down for a nap and sleep for hours but on other days she will lay down and only stay for a very few minutes. It is impossible to guess how her mind works. She was looking at a picture of her and several other women. She held up the picture and asked "who is this ugly one." At other times she will look at the same picture and not even recognize herself.

Showers always seem to be a traumatic time and hair shampooing is even worse. We have tried several different approaches in an effort to make it somewhat easier. Now, we sit her on the end of a transfer bench then must turn her 90 degrees. We then move her across the bench to the side of the bath tub. It is then necessary to lift her legs over the edge into the bath tub. The leg lifting seems to cause her significant pain in her right hip. She then must be moved to the far end of the transfer bench and positioned over the cut-out. After the shampoo and shower, the move out of the bath tub must be done in reverse. We have secured a new transfer bench which has a swivel seat and the seat slides. With this new bench she is sat on the seat with the cut-out, the seat is rotated 90 degrees and then is slid to the far side of the bath tub. Of course, her legs must be raised and placed in the bath tub. Initially this new transfer bench seems to be a significant improvement for both the patient and the person giving the shower.

She has always been a very neat and well organized person. Some days she still exhibits those traits but then there are days when her things are in complete disarray. She has sat at her table most of the afternoon and has been deeply involved in moving things around and arranging them in a neat and orderly way. Her empty golf ball boxes are filled with various small items but they are placed in the boxes in just a certain way. The boxes are carefully arranged to present a very organized appearance. She has placed her baby doll in a special location and I noted that the doll is now wearing a Kleenex diaper. She has placed the diaper on very carefully. The diaper on the front of the doll looks exactly the same as the diaper on the back side of the doll. The Kleenex diaper has no visible folds or creases on either side. Her day today was definitely one of those neat and very well organized days.

It is the Thanksgiving season and we celebrated one week early this year. Part of the family must travel several hundred miles and always stays in our home. They arrived later than planned on a Friday evening and so her bed time was over two hours later than usual. The next day, the day of celebration, was a good day for her and she remained alert and responsive all day. Her bed time was the normal time and she seemed to sleep well. She had trouble getting awake on the following day and after eating a small breakfast a five hour nap was in order. Again she had a problem getting fully awake but did eat an early dinner and then napped in her wheel chair until early evening. Then finally she was fully awake and responsive. There were problems with her taking her medication both in the morning and early evening. I'm sure the change in routine and the presence of guests for two days in a normally quiet environment contributed to some confusion. Hopefully today she will return to somewhat normal.

The official Thanksgiving Day was today. No cooking for us because we had a reservation at a nearby restaurant. They always serve outstanding food and we have always enjoyed visiting it. They had several menu choices but we chose the traditional Thanksgiving dinner and we shared. When they brought the main course, I was involved in splitting the meal and getting her plate ready. That wasn't soon enough because she took a fork and started eating off our son's plate. When the splitting was finished she was content to eat from her own plate. She ate a large dinner and when the dessert was served it was placed in front of my wife. I thought that would be easier for her to eat and I could just reach over when I wanted a bite. When I reached for the first bite, she immediately moved the small plate as far from me as possible. She ate her fill and it was indeed an enjoyable day.

I have been giving my Sweetheart chewing gum because she can't brush her own teeth. I recently discovered that the gum has an additional benefit for her. When she is upset if given a stick of gum, she calms right down. When the hospice people come to give her a shower she always gets upset when being undressing. Now, we just keep a small dish of gum in the bathroom. On shower day, she is wheeling into the bathroom, given a stick of gum and she sits calmly while being undressed, showered and dressed again after the shower.

And thus ended the fourth day.

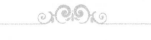

CHAPTER 5

The Fifth Day

And God said, Let the water bring forth abundantly the moving creature that hath life, and fowl that may fly above the earth in the open firmament of heaven. And God created great whales and every living creature that moveth, which the waters brought forth abundantly, after their kind, and every winged fowl after his kind: And God saw that it was good. And God blessed them, saying, Be fruitful, and multiply, and fill the waters in the seas, and let fowl multiply in the earth. Genesis 1:20-23

She sits in her wheel chair in our living room at her table which is loaded with her things. She spends hours arranging and rearranging so that the table has an orderly appearance. I am constantly in search of items that may be of interest which will keep her occupied. Our caregiver who comes two days each week recently brought a wooden basket which was fashioned to depict Noah's Ark. It was loaded with wooden animals which were cut from ¾ inch wood material and painted with appropriate colors. She tried to bite one of the wooden animals and exclaimed "that is hard as a rock!" She spends a significant amount of time handling the small animals.

As time goes by it seems that she is becoming more possessive. She doesn't want to be left in a room alone even for just a few minutes. She usually never notices that she is alone when she is fully engrossed at her table. When she does notice that she has been left alone, she immediately starts fussing, whining or crying. When you return, she always wants to know where you have been.

Today was a good day but then all days are good days. Some days are definitely better than others but that is to be expected. December has just arrived with cold and stormy weather. Taking her outside is no longer an option. The new shower transfer bench is in full use and is a tremendous improvement not only for the patient but also for the person giving the shower. The old transfer bench required significant effort while the new bench requires the same effort as helping her sit on the commode.

Giving medications is a simple process when the patient cooperates. Often that is not the case. Frequently the pill grinder must be put to use. I have tried several different methods to give the ground-up pills and the method of choice at this time is with juice. Nearly always she drinks her juice through a straw. I simply put the ground medication in the juice and let it settle to the bottom of the glass (no stirring). Then, I give her the juice to drink and the first few swallows sucks the medication off the bottom of the glass. No need for her to drink the full contents of the glass to get the medication.

My Sweetheart always did the cooking. The only thing that I ever cooked was limited to the barbeque. It wasn't that I couldn't cook but that was one of her many jobs. Now it is exclusively my job. She had hundreds of recipes but most were untried. Her favorites were usually gotten from other people and then she had improved upon them. One of her favorites was orange rolls. The original recipe came from my Mother and of course my Sweetheart made some improvements. She didn't rely on her memory but always reduced the recipes, with improvements, to writing.

I am constantly trying different recipes to find those that appeal to her. I like the recipes where we can have some leftovers so we can continue eating for several meals. About once each week is roasted chicken day. After the main meal, the remainder is deboned and we can eat chicken sandwiches. The last of the deboned chicken is then cut into small pieces and becomes chicken noodle soup, heavy on the noodles. A large pot of the chicken noodle soup will last for several meals.

She has no sense of taste but loves sweet foods. One of her favorites has always been frozen jam. I have been unable to find frozen jams in a grocery store so I have been forced to make it myself. Every few weeks I get a supply of the ingredients and spend part of a day making jam. It has always turned out successful and she enjoys it on toast and pancakes. The jam even tastes good to me.

I don't do well at house cleaning. My sweetheart always took care of that job and did it very well. Now it is my job. The kitchen is not an issue except for the tiled kitchen floor. It seems to get dirtier and dirtier but I just ignore it. I do OK with vacuuming but just don't seem to get around to dusting. When it comes to cleaning the toilets, they just don't get cleaned nearly as often as they should. I need to set aside one day of the week as toilet cleaning day.

She has a good appetite and usually eats well at each meal. It seems that she is becoming less and less capable of feeding herself. I find that she needs closely watched at meal times and fed some or most of every meal. She never complains of being hungry or thirsty but when a drink is offered, she will frequently drink the majority of a full glass of water or juice.

How are your sewing skills? My skills leave a lot to be desired. We have a sewing machine in our basement but I can't wind a bobbin, put in a wound bobbin, change threads or thread the sewing machine. I can sew a straight or zig-zag stitch when the machine is fully ready. Unfortunately there is no one around that can do what I can't pertaining to the sewing machine.

About 9 months ago it had become necessary to use trousers with an elastic waist for my wife. Several pairs of size 8P were purchased. They fit well, looked nice, and were easy to launder. She started gaining back some of the weight she had lost and soon it was necessary to buy some larger trousers in size 10P and then in size 14P. With the bulk from the pull up diapers we have found that size 18P is much easier for the caregiver. With each purchase it has become necessary to shorten the trouser legs and exercise my poor sewing skills. I just finished shortening two pair of trousers. Between struggling with my poor eye sight, shaky hands, finding a needle with an eye large enough that I could thread, the shortening turned into quite an ordeal. I'm sure that an examination of my work by a good seamstress would give her nightmares.

Christmas is less than one week away. We haven't been concerned with Christmas decorations for several years and this year is no different. My Sweetheart doesn't know that it is the Christmas season or even what Christmas is all about. She just lives day to day and seems to remain cheerful and pleasant. At times she will talk endlessly with her words making no sense but she enjoys talking. She frequently punctuates her talking with gestures and laughter. She is a joy to be with.

This being the Christmas season we can expect snow at various times during the winter months. We live on a small acreage and we have a huge asphalt driveway which is a significant problem when it comes to snow removal. We had a storm overnight and at 5:30 this morning I was shoveling. I normally only concentrate on an area in front of the garage and an area on a slight incline to enter the roadway. The mandatory shoveling was completed in about an hour and I had retired to the basement to read my newspaper. I heard a sound and immediately went upstairs to check and make sure my Sweetheart was OK. All was well so I retired back to the basement to continue my reading. Again I heard a sound and went back upstairs to check. Then, I noticed that a neighbor with a large tractor and scraper was involved in clearing my entire driveway. His efforts were sincerely appreciated.

As time goes by, she seems to sleep more and more. Sleepless nights are no longer of concern and usually she will sleep from 9 at night until 8 or 9 in the morning. She has started dozing more and more in her wheel chair and I will ask if she would like to lay on the bed and nap. She seems to always indicate that she does. Some days she will sleep for over 5 hours during the day. When night comes she is always ready to retire at the normal time. The Hospice nurse tells me that this is normal for people with dementia as they advance to the final stages. It is hard for me to accept that explanation but a person must just face the facts. Nothing that I can do will change that.

Some days she will only say a few words but on other days she will chatter almost constantly. On the talkative days they are just groups of words that convey no meaning. There are those rare days when a phrase is uttered and it makes complete sense. I was sitting in a folding chair at her side while she was diligently working at her table. I leaned over and whispered in her ear "I'm going to kiss you." She looked at me and immediately responded "I'm not easy." Frequently when she is asked if she would like a drink, she will respond "I don't drink." Most times when a question is asked she will not respond at all or if she does, her response will have nothing to do with the question.

Today in the local newspaper was a very long editorial which was titled "Nursing Care Call Unnerves Families." At this time over 1.5 million Americans are receiving care in assisted living or skilled nursing care facilities. The article expounds of the anguish that families face on making decisions concerning placement of family members in care facilities. I am very fortunate to not need to make those decisions. The placement of my Sweetheart in a care facility was never a consideration. Caring for her is not always easy but I view it as a privilege, not a burden.

The weather today was quite brisk and didn't get much over 35 degrees but it was a sunny day. It was a good day for a drive in the country. It is always a chore to move her from the house to the car and get the seat belt fastened. I dressed her in a heavy sweater and then wrapped her in a blanket. When she was in the car I covered her well until the heater had warmed the car. As soon as we started driving she was asking for her glasses which turn dark in the sunlight. She hasn't worn her glasses in months but a pair of sunglasses were in the car and she was content wearing them. We travelled the country roads for about an hour looking at the sights. She was alert and seemed to enjoy the change. When we returned home, it was difficult moving her from the car to the wheel chair and getting her inside but it was accomplished without incident. It was a good day for me and I believe it was an outstanding day for her. I'm sure it was a welcome change to the daily routine.

I just finished a period of over four weeks when I was the sole caregiver for 24 hours each day. My paid caregiver who comes 2 days each week for 7 hours each day, had just became a grandmother again and needed some time to do grandmother things. Then, with the holiday season upon us, she needed holiday time for herself and her family. During that 4 week span I only left our home 4 times for about 2 hours each time to shop for groceries. That 4 week period was a good wake up call to again make me realize the importance of having some help. We are so fortunate, myself and my Sweetheart, to have found someone to provide loving care. I well remember the day she was interviewed. She had no professional qualifications but she has a master's degree from practical experience. When I asked about her family her response was that she was the second child in a family of 13 children and that she had changed more diapers by the age of 12 than most women changed in a lifetime. Upon graduation from high school she provided care for her grandmother for a significant period of time. She is a mother of seven children of her own. Our caregiver is a lady with over 30 years of care giving practical experience. That kind of experience can't be learned in a classroom. She is an excellent cook and keeps us with a constant supply of cookies and brownies. She is an excellent seamstress and trims my Sweetheart's hair whenever it is needed.

I clearly remember our first visit to the neurologist and was told to get the book "A 36 Hour Day" and read it. I did and it has been very helpful. It has recently occurred to me that most books of this nature are written by professional medical personnel. I suggest that those professional personnel can address the medical aspects but the practical aspects of care giving can only be addressed by them based upon hearsay. There is a great deal of difference between the "school solution" and the real world practical application of care giving. There is no school solution. Each patient is different and each caregiver is different. There are literally hundreds of issues that must be addressed by the caregiver and each issue could have multiple solutions. The correct solution to an issue is the one that works best at the time with a particular patient and the caregiver. One never knows what solution works best unless various solutions have been tried and the results observed and evaluated. Care giving involves constantly searching for what works best. What works best today may not work best tomorrow.

She had just finished her shower when the telephone rang. The person calling asked to speak to my wife calling her by name. I immediately questioned her on who she was and why she was calling. I was informed it was someone from her doctor's office. I told her she could certainly speak to my wife but that she had dementia and probably wouldn't respond and if she spoke that her words would not have any meaning to her. The caller was apologetic and asked if I was her husband and that they had a request to refill a prescription. She went on to say that it had been over 9 months since her last doctor's visit and she should come in for re-evaluation. My response was that she could certainly come to see the doctor but that she had been under hospice care for over 9 months and I questioned the necessity for a visit. The caller again was very apologetic and said that the nurse apparently was not aware of her condition. Her regular doctor was off that day as was her nurse and one of the other doctors in the clinic was responding. It was apparent that they had not adequately reviewed her records before calling.

Today is her 75th birthday and the 319th day since she entered the hospice program. At the time she entered the program, I asked the doctor if that means she will die within 6 months. Her response was that she is just entering the program but no one knows how long that she will live. I gave her a birthday card this morning and it was really kind of a simple card except the front of the card was a brightly colored flower. Inside wasn't much of a verse and it was in rather small letters. I took a wide tipped pen and wrote in large letters various things for her thinking that she may be able to read them. One of the phrases that was written was "today you are 75 years old." I asked if she could read any of the things that I had written but she would only say a word now and then. When she came to the phrase that I had written she read "today you are old." She has spent a large amount of time just sitting and looking at the card. I think it is one of those days where periodically she will have flashes of reality and understanding. I'm sure that even though she can't read the words or phrases aloud that she knows and understands the meaning. We took her to lunch at one of her favorite places. When we were leaving the restaurant, we had some difficulty getting her back into the car. She was almost dropped to the pavement but she remained quite calm during the whole ordeal. After arrival back at our home, she was given some small toys and a bouquet of flowers. She loved the small toys and when the flowers were delivered she showed some excitement. She had an opportunity to talk with the family members who could not be with her in person. She listened to them and was quite talkative. I believe that this birthday was one of the best ever. It may not be remembered by her but it was truly a memorable day for those family members at home and afar.

My Sweetheart had visitors today. In fact she had several who came at various times. It was interesting to watch as the different visitors came because it seemed that the more that came, the more she talked. She was talking and laughing constantly. The last visitors came a short time before her normal bedtime. She was still laughing and talking but when she was laid down on the hospital bed she was asleep immediately. It was a very good day for her.

She usually does well feeding herself but there are days when she doesn't do well at all. Then there are days like today at lunch time. I fixed her a plate with ½ of a roasted chicken sandwich, potato chips, some small sweet pickles, and some orange pineapple jello. I made sure that the jello was mixed enough that it could be easily eaten with a spoon. I gave her the plate and a teaspoon but she wanted to eat everything on her plate using the teaspoon. Needless to say, it doesn't work well to eat a sandwich, potato chips or pickles. I attempted to give her some assistance but she was not interested. She continued eating with the spoon until the plate was clean to include the sandwich. It was a little frustrating to watch and certainly not the normal way of eating a sandwich, potato chips or pickles but it worked for her and that's what is important.

Her normal sleeping pattern now is 12-13 hours at night and then a 3-5 hour nap during the day. That is a lot of sleep. During her waking hours she is either eating or sitting at her table with her toys. When she talks, she always talks in low tones. At no time can I remember when she has raised her voice. I believe that you can tell how a person feels by the strength of their voice. I don't mean how loud or soft but there is some quality in a voice that gives it strength. There is very little strength in her voice. She has always been concerned about her appearance and regardless of the time of day or night, when she is wheeled past a mirror she is checking and rearranging her hair so she looks presentable. She still has a large wardrobe but only wears a few items of clothing. Her normal attire is trousers with an elastic waist and a pull-over shirt or blouse. Being in a wheel chair she seldom wears slippers but is just in stocking feet. The slippers seem to cause a problem with constantly slipping all or partially off.

Yes, I firmly believe that regardless of how severe the dementia that a few times each day the fog may clear and they will be a recollection of current and past events. Today was a day when that belief was somewhat confirmed. She had just finished her mid-day nap and was wheeled out to her table. When she saw a small baby doll she exclaimed "Oh, it's my baby girl!" Then, she thought for a minute and said "Oh, that's not mine, I have baby boys." She had three boys. They are grown now but they were her baby boys.

It is a Thursday and the time is 4 AM with no sleep until now. This seems to be a repeat of last Monday early morning. I woke from a sound sleep at 2 AM and it was apparent that she needed changing. She had spent the entire night tossing and turning but after the BM she slept soundly. Monday and Tuesday nights were very similar in that she seemed to sleep well during the night, usually 12 to 13 hours. During the daytime she would nap for normally 4 to 5 hours. Then there was Wednesday night. In bed at 8:30 PM and asleep immediately for an hour and then nothing but tossing and turning. Finally at 11 PM she had her first BM since Monday then more tossing and turning. I changed her several times in hopes that would make it possible for her to rest. She would lay and mutter, kicking off the bed coverings and partially removing her diaper. It was apparent that without bed coverings she would never sleep. Finally in desperation, I pulled the sheet and blanket up to her chin and then firmly attached them to the railings on each side of the bed. She tugged at them for a short period of time and finally at 4 AM sleep arrived. I believe that we are both completely exhausted.

We have always tried to keep our affairs in order. Before the dementia had progressed to the advanced stages, we established a family trust, new wills, powers of attorney and several other legal documents. I recently became aware of a nearby Federal Credit Union that was offering certificates of deposit with an interest rate four times higher than any other financial institutions. Needless to say, I moved some money. My wife's Social Security had been deposited at another Federal Credit

Union for years. I wanted to close that account and change her Social Security deposit to a different Federal Credit Union. I gathered all of the necessary information and went to the local Social Security office to make the change. I told the agent the purpose for my visit and showed him the Power of Attorney that permitted me to act in her behalf. His response was that Social Security does not recognize the Power of Attorney because it is a State document. He then asked if she could come into the office and sign her own name and answer some questions. I responded that although she was bedridden, I could bring her into the office but she could no longer sign her name and doesn't understand when questions are asked. He proceeded to ask me some questions and obtain my signature through electronic authentication. He then said they would send some information to her doctor to verify her condition and that the change should be forthcoming. Today she received a letter explaining some information and giving her the right to appeal my designation as her representative. The letter and a pamphlet outlined a requirement for me to make periodic reports to Social Security on how her money was spent. I just wanted to change where it was deposited to make things easier but now I seem to have created a monster for myself and made things more difficult. But looking on the bright side, I have a new title, I'm now a "Representative Payee."

Last night she slept and she slept well. She was in bed at 8:30 PM and woke at 9:30 AM the next morning. After a light breakfast she was napping in her wheel chair so she was laid in her bed. She slept soundly for over 5 hours and then was awoke for an early dinner. She never seemed to get fully awake but continued to nap in her wheel chair. I tried and tried to get her awake but to no avail. The time for her night medications was fast approaching. In desperation I got a small bowl of ice cream and started to feed her about a half hour before medication time. Each bite seemed to hasten her awakening. After her last bite of ice cream, the night medication was placed in her hand and she swallowed it without hesitation. I will remember this and I'm sure the same system will be used again sometime in the future.

Today was the day when we were going to lunch at a very nice restaurant. The plans were made the night before and we intended to leave home about 11 AM. At 8 AM the weather turned bad and the snow started. I gave her a small breakfast and promptly at 11 AM we migrated to the car with her in a coat and covered with a blanket. We just had her seated in the car when I noted a bad smell. Back into the house and she was changed and then back to the car. The roads were not terrible in spite of the snow and when we arrived at the restaurant we noted that not many cars were in the parking lot. We picked a space very close to the restaurant and moved her out of the car and into the wheel chair. Just before we arrived at the front door of the restaurant we were informed that the restaurant was closed for kitchen remodeling. We went back to the car and loaded her in again. We decided to go to a different restaurant which was close by. Upon arriving at the next restaurant we noted a handicapped parking spot right in front but before we could park another car took the parking spot. We circled the restaurant and the only parking spot was on the street at the side of the restaurant but there was a large curb on the passenger side which made wheel chair access almost impossible. We backed into the spot facing the wrong direction but at least the wheel chair access was now on the passenger side which made it workable. We off loaded and enjoyed a nice lunch. When dessert was served she was in a finger eating mode and at times it became quite messy but she enjoyed the pie. The return home was uneventful. In spite of some of the problems the outing was enjoyable.

Nothing seems to be constant. Something that has worked for a considerable period of time may no longer be effective or it may be effective on some days and not on other days. It seems that care giving is a never ending process of trial and error. Some things have been tried several times without success but now they are successful. The only thing that is constant is change.

She wears a narcotic pain patch because of her non-functional right hip which gives her significant pain. The narcotic pain patch needs to be changed every third day. Today was day number three and in the process of changing the patch, the old patch could not be found. I carefully search the area where they are always applied but the old patch could not be located. The caregiver informed me that she had found the old pain patch and it was attached to her underclothing. She showered the day before and the patch was attached when the shower was completed. There is no way to tell how long she has been without the pain patch. Looking back, it seems that she has been more alert in the few hours which may be an indication that she has been without the pain patch for a fairly significant period of time. I do not routinely check to see if the patch is attached but do note it's presence from time to time. I need to change my ways and check periodically throughout the day.

It seems there are always things that can be done differently to make life better for both the patient and the caregiver. When she is in the wheel chair, she is usually wears trousers or a skirt, both of which require additional effort when she is being dressed. Our hired caregiver that comes two days each week suggested that we may want to consider doing something a little different. She suggested taking a housecoat which buttons, zips or snaps in front and while she is sitting in the wheel chair slip it on her backwards. That way it would cover her in front and on the legs and can be tucked in securely at the sides. She went on to say that the housecoat could be trimmed or slit at the top and in the back so it would be a better fit. She was 100% correct. It was tried today and it fits well, is comfortable for the patient and is much easier for the caregiver.

We live on a two acre lot with a large front lawn and the back acre is our private forest with pine trees over 50 feet tall. The pines are a variety of species with some being the long needle variety. Most of the trees shed their old pine needles each winter, consequently, the entire area needs raking in the late winter or early spring. Almost daily I will go to the forest and rake piles of pine needles. When the air quality index is acceptable, the piles of needles are burned. I was nearly finished with my yearly raking task and about 5 PM had fired the last four piles of pine needles. I watched them burn until the flames were almost gone and the remains were just smoldering. About 7 PM that evening, a knock came to our door and when I opened the door I was confronted by a large fireman who wanted to know if I had been burning something. I told him that I had and that it was legal for me to burn. He went on to say that some of the neighbors had complained about the smoke and wanted to know if I could extinguish the fire. I told him it was just smoldering but I certainly would. All the while the fire engine was parked in our driveway with all lights on and flashing. I definitely need to rake and burn the needles each year but I surely don't need that kind of attention.

I always try to do things the same way. It is my belief that being consistent makes things much easier for the patient. The routine at bed time is that the wheel chair is moved to the side of the hospital bed. She is assisted to a standing position, her trousers are lowered and then she is sat on the side of the hospital bed. Then, she is again assisted to a standing position, the diaper is removed and she is sat on the bedside commode. A clean pull up diaper is then put onto her legs and pulled up to her knees. She is again assisted to the standing position, the clean diaper is pulled up and she is sat back on the side of the hospital bed then laid on the bed and covered. During the process last evening while helping her out of the wheel chair to the standing position, she bit me on the chest. I don't have a clue as to why but apparently she just thought it was the right thing to do. I hope that doesn't happen often.

Today is anniversary day. One year ago today she was inducted into the hospice program. Looking back there have been many changes in the last year and I'm sure there will be many more changes. Today was an unusual day and maybe there will be more days like this in the future. I woke her at 8:15 AM so she could be given her morning medications and breakfast before the paid caregiver arrived because this was an off day for me. All went well until it was time for breakfast. She would not drink any liquids and took only one bite of food. I tried several different things but without success. She just refused to eat or drink and sat in her wheel chair dozing. At 9 AM she was put into her hospital bed and was asleep immediately. She remained in bed sleeping until three in the afternoon. She did eat a good meal when she awoke but it was a one meal day.

Today was the beginning of a new year. This is day 366 on hospice and as I reflect back during this past year there have been 5 nights when I was away from my sweetheart. Three of those nights she was in a care facility which was not a good experience. The remaining two nights she was here in our home and our two day each week caregiver stayed and provided care. That worked very well. Many things have changed but not many have been for the best but every day is filled with memories that will be cherished.

Several times each week we receive magazines or small catalogs. They usually end up on her work table and she looks at the pages, tears out the pages, tears up the pages and often folds them carefully. Tonight she was looking at a magazine and had torn out some pages. She had parts of two pages that she was looking at carefully. I made some comment for her to giving me the papers so I could put them into the waste basket. She responded no that she wanted to read them. I asked her what was written on the pages and her response was "WORLD BEAT" and "NOT OVER". I really didn't understand and looked at the pages. Printed at the top of the two pages were those exact words in bold letters.

How much weight can you lift? As I get older, I struggle with anything over 40 pounds. I am involved with lifting my wife several times each day. When she is lifted, she usually plants her left foot and I lift and pull her forward until she is in a standing position. She is then just rotated 90 degrees and seated on the bed, on the commode or in the wheel chair. Today is her third day with no BM and I am quite concerned. This evening I took her to the bathroom in hopes that sitting on the toilet rather than the commode would help stimulate a BM. As usual, I lifted and pulled her forward to the standing position and started to lower her trousers. Then disaster, her left leg gave away and there was no way that I could hold her. She slid to the bathroom floor and was laying full length on the floor. Hospice people have said that when a patient falls that 911 should be called and the closest agency will respond with assistance. Before calling I wanted to make her more comfortable so she was assisted in moving to a sitting position. I moved behind her, slid my hands and arms under her armpits and lifted until she could be seated on the toilet. She weighs 145 pounds and there is no way that I can lift that much weight, but I did. I won't try it again.

Her sleeping habits appear to be changing but there seems to be no set pattern. Most nights she will sleep uninterrupted for 12 to 14 hours. Some days she will nap from 3 to 7 hours but there are also days with no naps at all. Today was a 7 hour nap day. After the long nap she was alert and fully engrossed in working at her table. She had a small new clothing catalog and was diligently looking at the colorful pages. Some pages were torn out of the catalog and were carefully folded. She picked up a hand held mirror and was studying the image when she exclaimed "that is my friend." She made that same remark several times during the evening.

Things are constantly changing but I am a little slow making changes. In the past it became a habit to put things away and never leave anything lying in sight because my Sweetheart would move it and then forget where it was placed. I am constantly catching myself in the process of moving something which I don't want her to touch. I seem to forget that the only way she can get her hands on any object is with my assistance. It is late afternoon and about two hours before time for her evening medications. I brought the medications into the kitchen and laid them on the cabinet and the thought stuck me that I should move them out of sight. Then I realized no need to move them because she can't reach them unless I assist. I guess it is a constant effort for me to be retrained.

I order her pull up diapers from the internet and through trial and error have found what works best for us. We like the Tena brand heavy protection super plus underwear. At the beginning, we followed the chart and ordered S/M which fits waist size 29-40 but they were too difficult to put on. We then ordered the Large which fits 37-50 and we were very satisfied with them but there was also some difficulty in getting them pulled up. By mistake, the last order was for size XL. The error wasn't noticed until I opened a package and then my mistake was obvious. However, the XL size may be even better because they are very easily pulled up. They do fit a little looser but the jury is still out as to whether they are the preferred size.

I often have to feed her but there are times when she feeds herself and does very well. I have tremors and sometimes the feeding becomes a two handed operation. Lunch today was a sandwich, pickle slices and chips. I put the pickle slices on a saucer and laid a fork beside it. She ate the pickle slices with her fingers. Then, she ate the sandwich and chips with the fork. That is not an easy task but she was able to do it quite well. It seems that sometime during every meal she has an urge to pour her drink into her plate of food. When she has eaten her fill she will put her napkin in the glass with the remaining drink. She definitely makes meal time interesting.

Old habits are hard to break for all of us. Last evening my Sweetheart was sitting at her table working diligently on folding papers, placing them carefully on the table and rearranging everything. I noticed that she was constantly pulling small pieces of straw from one of her baskets. She finally was able to get one of the pieces which was about the size of a toothpick. She immediately put it into her mouth and started picking her teeth. I offered to dispose of it in the garbage but she resisted saying that she was using it. She continued using it as a toothpick for several minutes and when she was finished she asked me to throw it into the garbage. Before the onset of dementia she always had a good supply of toothpicks and was constantly using them.

We have a small formal dining room. The dining room table sits in the center directly under the chandelier. Today the table was moved away from the full length windows that look out across our back yard and into our own private forest. This morning she was positioned in front of the full length picture window in the dining area and she sat for the longest time enjoying the view. She looked and looked at the view of the forest. When asked if she remembered walking in the forest and working in the garden, a sparkle came into her eyes. I'm sure for just an instant her memory was clear and she did remember.

It is getting more and more difficult for her to take her medications. The morning medications are now crushed and sprinkled on toast covered with freezer jam. One of the night medications is a small pill that can't be crushed. Last night that one pill was put inside a hollowed out piece of caramel popcorn and a little soft butter was applied to hold the pill in place. The piece of popcorn was then marked with a small red mark using strawberry jam. She took the pill with no problem along with other pieces of caramel corn. Undoubtedly she chewed it some before swallowing which is not desirable but in this case it was necessary.

Fifty six years ago she worked in a small town drug store. In those days every small town had a drug store or two or three. Each drug store had a soda fountain which served soft drinks, ice cream and milk shakes. I frequently went to the drug store while she was working and she would make chocolate milk shakes for me. Tonight I decided to make her a chocolate milk shake using half vanilla ice cream and half rocky road. I poured it into an old fashioned coke cola glass with the small bottom making it easier for her to hold. Her first swallow she exclaimed "this is good!" Then another swallow and "this tastes great!" I could see the joy in her face as she savored every swallow.

At times she will sit at her table and be fully engrossed in what she is doing. There are other times when her thoughts seem to be in some distant place at another time. I never know what person is going to show up for the day or the evening. Last evening she sat at her table and she seemed extremely alert and attentive. She seemed to be aware of what was happening around her. At one point she picked up her small doll and cradled it in her arms and looked intently into its eyes. Then in a soft voice she exclaimed "you are a cute little terd." I was somewhat shocked but couldn't help smiling.

When is she awake and when is she asleep? That should be readily apparent but is not always the case. There are times when I will enter the bedroom and she will be lying in bed with her eyes wide open. As I move around the room her eyes never waiver from staring at the ceiling. I can stand next to the bed and move directly above her but the gaze never waivers. She will blink her eyes regularly as she stares. If not disturbed she will soon close her eyes and there is no doubt that she has been asleep the entire time.

The morning oral medications are two tablets and one capsule. Each morning the contents of the capsule are sprinkled on buttered toast along with the two crushed tablets. A generous portion of freezer jam is then spread on the toast and the slice is quartered. She eats the toast with the medications without hesitation. The night oral medications are again two tablets and one capsule. One of the tablets is timed release and is not to be ground. I have experimented with many different ways in getting her to take the night medications. One of the latest was with prunes. I sliced the prunes in half and inserted one tablet into each half then the prunes were dropped in a small dish of caramel popcorn. All went well until she started chewing the first prune and when she felt the tablet in her mouth the partially eaten prune was spit out. That same thing happened with the other half of the prune. My latest effort and I hope my last was back to the old standby, toast and jam. The timed release tablet was cut in half and inserted into the toast and again the generous portion of freezer jam. She ate the whole thing without hesitation. I think it is time to stop experimenting.

Today was a very good day. One of our sons came in the late afternoon. When he came through the door there was instant recognition. She didn't know for sure who he was but she did know that he was family. During his visit she was very happy, smiling and often laughing. A short time later we snapped some pictures while she was laughing. As the visit ended she gave him a hug and with a big smile said "Thanks for coming."

Sometimes I shop on the internet. It saves travel, time and money with the goods being delivered to our door. The downside is that we receive lots of solicitations. Weekly we receive several small catalogs for clothing and household goods. These small catalogs are placed on my sweethearts work table. She spends hours looking at the catalogs, tearing out the pages and carefully folding them. She seldom looks at them after the pages have been removed from the catalog. Each morning I look over her work table and remove some of the clutter. She no longer has much interest in the small wooden animals but occasionally will remove them from one of her baskets but soon goes back to her catalog pages.

Today was a very different day. The normal for several weeks has been sleeping from 13 to 15 hours each night and then napping for 2 to 4 hours during the day. Last night she slept only 12 ½ hours and there was no napping during the day. She was alert and talkative. She looked through a picture album and recognized our children and called them by name. She also recognized grandchildren and named their father. When she would see a picture of an old friend or school mate, she was able to recall their name in some instances. When she is asked a question, she rarely gives a response. Today when I asked how she was doing the response was "Oh, so so." This was one of the few days when her thinking seemed quite clear.

I don't hear well. In fact I have hearing aids but am not in the habit of wearing them. As time has passed I've noticed that I have more and more trouble hearing and understanding people. In the past few weeks I have made a concerted effort to wear the hearing aids during all of my waking hours. Today I noticed that the hearing aid in my right ear seemed to have a distant chirping sound. I determined that the cause was a weak battery and so new ones were installed. The chirping sound seemed to continue so I then removed the hearing aids and decided they must need repairing. After they were removed I noticed the chirping sound continued so my next thought was that I needed an appointment with an ENT doctor. A little later in the day some people came to our house to visit and immediately asked what was making that chirping sound. After doing some checking it was determined that it was from the carbon monoxide detector warning of low batteries. I replaced the batteries but never breathed a word of what had transpired before the people arrived. The next morning I noticed the chirping sound again and assumed the new battery that I had installed was a faulty battery. Having one new battery left, I removed the old one and installed the new one. In the process I noted that the new battery package indicated that it should be used before 2002 and it is now 2014. Needless to say, that battery doesn't work either. I couldn't even figure out such a simple thing and just think, I'm the caregiver.

Today was one of those rare days. It started quite normally with a shower and a little later in the day she napped for about 2 hours. After the nap, she was extremely alert. Most days when she talks, it has no meaning because it is just a bunch of words that don't relate. Today when she was asked a question, she would respond with an answer that had meaning. Later in the day our youngest son visited. She definitely recognized him and at one point, she looked at him and said "I love you." When he was preparing to leave she looked at him and said "thanks for coming to visit me." It was definitely a day when her mind seemed clear and a day to be remembered.

And thus ended the fifth day.

CHAPTER 6

The Sixth Day

A nd God said, Let the earth bring forth the living creature after his kind, cattle and creeping thing, and beast of the earth after his kind: and it was so. And God made the beast of the earth after his kind, and cattle after their kind, and every thing that creepeth upon the earth after his kind: and God saw that it was good. And God said, Let us make man in our image, after our likeness: and let them have dominion over the fish of the sea, and over the fowl of the air, and over the cattle, and over all the earth, and over every creeping thing that creepeth upon the earth. So God created man in his own image, in the image of God created he him; male and female created he them. ***** Genesis 1:24-27.

She has now been a hospice patient for 16 months. She seems to be quite stable and has a good appetite. The hospice nurse informed me during her last visit that she may change her visitation from twice each week to only one visit each week with the option for more visits when necessary. She also indicated that with her condition somewhat stabilized that it could be possible sometime in the future that she would need to be removed from the hospice program. The biggest problem if she were removed from the program would be with showers. When she is showered it is much easier if two people are assisting her. The undressing, movement into and out of the bathtub, the drying and the dressing become quite labor intensive and is difficult for one person to accomplish. Whatever happens will happen and we will have to adjust accordingly.

The paid caregiver said today that "this was her grateful day." I thought about that for a few minutes and wasn't sure that I understood. She said whenever she gave her anything, food, drink or anything else, she always said "Thank You." Additionally, when she was told "Thank You" her response was always "Your Welcome." It was a good day.

It is interesting to watch her and what she does and how she does it. She was sitting at the table eating and wanted a drink. I always keep a flexible straw in her glass but she frequently does not use it. She reached for her glass and the straw was pointed away. She took the glass and gradually rotated it until the straw was easily accessible and then lifted the glass and drank. She has her own way of doing things and at this time of life trying to change is not an option.

She sits at her table and at times appears to be trying to clean things. She takes some object and starts lightly rubbing the pages of a catalog or magazine. She will do the same thing on toys and other items. She becomes completely engrossed with her work and will sit for hours just rubbing away. She seems to get personal satisfaction from her efforts.

Memorial Day weekend arrived and I made my annual trek to the area where I was raise for a reunion with my siblings. My Sweetheart remained at home and was cared for by our caregiver. During my absence my thoughts were nearly always at home. I was never concerned about her welfare because I knew that she would be well cared for. I departed on Friday morning and returned before noon on Sunday. It was a good reunion but of course there was definitely something missing, my Sweetheart. Upon my return there was no sign of recognition when I entered our home. She was just living in her own world and seemed quite content in doing so.

The Hospice nurse asked me today what changes I had noted in her condition. I responded that I see her every day and any changes are so gradual that they don't seem apparent. There definitely have been changes. Her medications are not given in a pill form but are always ground, sprinkled on toast and covered with freezer jam. She seems to sleep much longer with some days being 18 hours or more. She does not talk nearly as much and when she does it often has no meaning. She will often speak the same word several times with no other words preceding or following. She is less cooperative at times especially during the evening hours. She seems to have a more difficult time standing even when she is assisted to the standing position. I need to do better in observing her and noticing change.

My Sweetheart has been taking a time released sleeping medication for many months but it seems there has been a drastic price increase. The Hospice nurse approached me about trying the same medication but not time released. I had on hand some of the medication we were going to try and after examining the prescription bottle, it indicated that it should be destroyed if not used by the end of November. It is June and no current medication was readily available so I have been using the outdated medication. It appears to be working just as well as the time released. I'm sure that we will get a new and current prescription and discontinue using the time released medication.

I laid her down for a nap at 12:30 PM today and she slept less than one hour. I changed her and put her into the wheel chair and as we were leaving the bedroom she said "let's get out of here." That was a good excuse to put her into the car and go for a drive in the country. We ended up at a nice restaurant in a town about 10 miles to the west of our home. The lunch was very good and she thoroughly enjoyed it. As we returned and drove into our driveway, she looked at our home and exclaimed "I love my house." She spent the evening sitting at her table, playing with her things, and constantly laughing and talking.

Today was my play day and I ventured out to a local golf course. My play days are sacred days and I refuse to have them interrupted for anything that can be addressed at another time. It was a good day on the golf course and as I was nearing home, I decided that I had just enough time for a haircut. About then my cell phone rang and it was my caregiver. She said that she was just putting in a load of washing when she noticed the floor drain in the utility room was overflowing. No haircut today. I rushed home and shut off everything that could add to the problem and called a local septic pumping business. They informed me that they provided service around the clock but it would be a little after 5 before the truck would arrive. I went out with a shovel and started probing for the location of the lid to the septic tank and was unable to find the exact location. The truck arrived and they found the lid and started pumping. About the time the truck arrived, my Sweetheart awoke from her nap so she was put at her table in the front room. The caregiver was vacuuming up water with a water vacuum and another technician was cleaning the drain lines. What could have ended up being a real disaster was at least mitigated to some degree. Sure, there is a mess but that can be cleaned up. The fans are going drying the carpet that was drenched and all of the plumbing facilities are now in working order. The haircut will have to wait for another day.

This was grocery shopping day. I had an offer from one of the ladies in our church to come and stay while I shopped. It was the same lady that cancelled another time 7 minutes before she was scheduled to arrive. Needless to say, I declined the offer. I am of the opinion that I just need to take care of things myself and not rely on any assistance. It is a real effort to grocery shop by pushing a wheel chair with one hand and pull a grocery cart with another but it can be done. One of the items purchased today was fresh cherries. I rinsed them well and started removing the pits when my sweetheart popped a cherry into her mouth. I was concerned about the cherry pit. No need for concern because she ate the cherry and put the pit on a Kleenex. Just to make sure that she didn't swallow a pit, I removed them from the other cherries before she ate them.

Morning and night medications are given on toast covered with jam so of course we use a lot of jam. I am constantly making another batch. In an effort to keep her weight down, I have been experimenting with making low sugar or no sugar jams. I recently made a batch of no sugar jam and it was a horrible failure. It was very thin and runny but it makes a fair topping. My sweetheart doesn't really care for bananas but I can slice one up and cover it with the failed no sugar jam and she will eat every bite. Today I made another batch of jam with a small amount of sugar, about 1/6 of the normal recipe. The jury is still out but I think that I may have a winner. I need to leave it sitting overnight and then put it in the freezer before I do the test.

The Hospice nurse came today to check a rash that my sweetheart has on the inside of her right arm. She called and confirmed that she believes it is SHINGLES – again for the second time. The pharmacy delivered the medication during late afternoon. It is Acyclovir 800 mg (horse pills). She is to take 1 tablet 5 times each day. I did some testing after the pills arrived. I ground one and tasted the powder which didn't appear to taste bitter. I mixed the one ground tablet with 4 ounces of her calorie free drink and the taste was not objectionable. I have a container which holds 16 ounces and is marked for each ounce. I ground a total of 4 tablets and put in the container. My instructions for the caregiver tomorrow will be to have my sweetheart consume 16 ounces of the drink with the ground tablets mixed in. Tonight I gave her a small dish of ice cream and sprinkled one ground tablet over the top. She ate all of the ice cream without hesitation. I prepared a large bowl of buttered popcorn for her to eat throughout the day to assist in getting her to drink the medication mixture. The caregiver was successful in getting all 16 ounces consumed and the ice cream worked the second time. It appears there will be no problem in getting all of the shingles medication taken as prescribed.

When the shingles medication was delivered, I did not receive any information concerning side effects and other items of concern. After checking on the internet for side effect information, the list was long and seemed to be all inclusive. The bottom line was the medication can cause almost every side effect except death was not listed. This morning she looked at me and asked "Who are you?" She hasn't asked that question in a long time. Is it a side effect of the medication or just normal progression of dementia? I guess it really doesn't matter.

When night time comes we have a regular ritual that takes place. At 7:30 she is given the night meds on a half slice of toast covered with jam. About 8:15 she seems to be getting rather sleepy so I take her into the bedroom to get her ready for bed. I remove her trousers and diaper, then sit her on the commode. I put on a clean diaper, lay her in bed and cover her with a sheet and blanket. Then the side railings are raised so she won't fall out of bed. I have had hearing aids for several years but only wore them on special occasions. For the last several months I have had more and more difficulty hearing so the hearing aids are being worn nearly all day every day. I remove them when I'm working and playing golf. It is amazing the difference in the volume on the TV with hearing aids as compared to no hearing aids. Tonight during our nightly ritual of course I was wearing my hearing aids. As I was assisting my sweetheart off the commode, one of the hearing aids popped out and fell into the commode. It was easy to find but did take a bit of effort. I don't think I want that to happen again.

Today was a strange day. She normally sleeps until after 11 AM unless it is necessary to wake her. This morning she woke at 7:30 and was not interested in sleeping after she was changed. By 9:30 she was dozing in her wheel chair and was laid down for a nap. The nap lasted only about one hour and then she was alert, talkative, smiling and laughing for the rest of the day.

The Social Worker came today for her monthly visit. She is concerned about my sweetheart but really seems more concerned about me, the caregiver. She is constantly checking to make sure that I take time away from caregiving and do some of the things that I like to do. She made a statement today that was very true but I had never thought of it in that manner. My role has gradually changed. In the early stages of dementia I was the husband giving care to his wife. As the disease has progressed, I became less of a husband and more of a caregiver. Does that make sense? I'm not sure but one needs to give that some deep thought because it really is true.

One of her medications is given to make her more cooperative. She is normally given a 5 mg tablet each morning and again each evening. On shower days she is given an extra 5 mg tablet just before the shower and it seems to help. I needed to cut her toe nails so she was given an extra 5 mg tablet and the toe nail cutting went well. It seems that on those days when she is given the extra tablet that she is more alert and talkative. The prescription indicates that she can be given no more than two of the extra 5 mg tablets each day. There never has been an instance when she was given more than one extra. It is my intent to give her an extra 5 mg tablet every morning and see if it has a lasting positive effect for the day.

She was alert and talkative most of the day today so the extra 5 mg tablet seems to be working. She talked a lot and was engrossed in her activities at her table. When night comes torn pages of magazines and catalog are scattered everywhere. It almost looks like a ticker tape parade route. Most of her talk has no meaning but occasionally she utters a phrase that is very pertinent to the time and place. Tonight I sidled up to her and gave her a kiss and told her that I loved her. She looked at me and responded "That's Good."

In the past it has been difficult to keep her covered during the night. I would wake frequently and would need to rearrange the sheet and blanket so that she was covered. There were times that it became necessary to tie the sheet and blanket so they could not be removed. This has all changed. She is normally put into bed between 8 and 8:30 each night. She is laid in the bed, covered and is asleep immediately. When she awakes 12-15 hours later her position in the bed is exactly the same as when she first went to sleep. Each time that I enter the room I look to make sure she is still breathing. There are times that I stand for several minutes before it is possible to detect any movement.

Our middle son came to town for our annual golf tourney. We picked him up at the airport and although my Sweetheart did not know his name it was obvious from the start that there definitely was recognition. All our sons were together with us for Chinese food and she ate, and ate, and ate. It was a buffet and when it seemed that she had finished, she would spot some other food item and eat until it was gone. At one point, I unwrapped a set of chopsticks and thought that she would enjoy playing with them. Not so, she spotted a piece of some kind of cake and immediately started eating it with chopsticks. She didn't use the chopsticks in the conventional way but used them as kind of a spoon and scooped the cake. I tried to replace the chopsticks with a conventional eating utensil but she was content using the chopsticks.

She sleeps very soundly at night and hardly moves. When I get out of bed in the morning I always stand and look at her to see if there is any movement. Before she awakes in the mornings I will visit the bedroom several times and always stand and look to make sure she is breathing.

I know someday that won't be the case. I hope than when she does go that she will go peacefully but of course I have no control over that.

Most days she sits at her table and is not responsive to questions or comments. On the rare occasions when she does respond, her response has no meaning. Then there are the times when her response is very pertinent and to the point. One of our sons was visiting and had spent several hours at our home. He was getting ready to leave and told his Mother that he had to leave now but he would come back. She looked at him and said "why"? A little later in the evening she was sitting and staring straight ahead. I asked "how are you?" She immediately responded with "I don't know?" One of our children had given her a small stuffed animal. She reached out to its tail and exclaimed "I love my dog." We received a piece of mail addressed to her in bold letters. When I gave it to her, her response was "Oh my goodness." I gave her a small dish of ice cream and she immediately took the spoon and exclaimed "That is what I want." Those times will surely be remembered.

Today was grocery shopping day. I loaded her into the car with her wheel chair and we went to a local grocery store. Naturally all of the handicapped parking spots were full and I definitely noted some of the patrons had undoubtedly pirated the handicapped tags. Grocery shopping isn't easy when one pushes a wheel chair with one hand and pulls a grocery cart with another but we did get the shopping done. It is a bag your own grocery store and it doesn't present any significant problem unless other customers bag their groceries with their carts parked in the middle of the walk way rather than at the end. When that happens it is even more difficult for other customers to dodge their grocery baskets. We left the store and went to our car at the far end of the parking lot. I needed to put my sweetheart into the car, store the wheel chair in the trunk and then unload the grocery cart into the trunk also. Just as I finished putting her into the car, an acquaintance had observed us leaving the grocery store and came across the parking lot to give us some assistance. It was not necessary at the time but it was sincerely appreciated. As we left the parking lot there were cars coming and we needed to find a space where we could merge into the traffic. Just as a space was approaching, my sweetheart exclaimed "Go, Go." It was apparent that at that particular moment she was well aware of her surroundings and what we needed to do to safely enter the main road.

The Hospice nurse suggested that with the amount of sleep that she has been getting that there may be no need to continue giving her the sleeping medication. She asked that I do some experimenting for a few days without giving her the medication. The first and second nights she slept very well but she awoke about 2 hours earlier than normal. The third night again she slept well and awoke the next morning at about the normal time. There have been some minor issues that may or may not be associated with the discontinued use of the sleep medication but I'm convinced that medicine is no longer required.

I frequently put her into the car and we run an errand or just go for a drive. It is interesting to note that although she doesn't understand many things that she does remarkably well in getting into and out of the car. There are certain things that she needs to do to make the entry and exit easier for both of us. It seems that she is able to recall those things and do them at just the right time. I'm sure that as time goes by her ability to do those things will also disappear.

I returned in the late afternoon from my day off. Of course, I had been on the golf course where I spend most of my leisure time. When I entered the room there was immediate recognition. Then, she exclaimed "happy birthday". It wasn't anyone's birthday but apparently she had that thought enter her mind just briefly. I questioned her on the birthday remark but could get no further response.

We had someone coming from our church today and was scheduled to arrive at 2:30 PM. That is her normal afternoon nap time. I decided that I would let her sleep longer than normal and then she would be awake and alert during the visit. At 1 PM she was still sleeping soundly but needed to be awaken. All went well during the visit but a short time after his departure, she was sleepy and laid down for an afternoon nap that lasted over 2 hours. Her total sleep for the 24 hour period was 19 hours. It seems that she wants to sleep more and more as time goes by.

Last week we were informed that our regular Hospice nurse will be leaving. The new nurse came with the regular nurse so she could get acquainted with the patient and the caregiver. The next visit was the regular nurse's final visit and there was a different replacement nurse when they came. It seems that the original replacement nurse had decided that she wasn't going to work there any longer. The new replacement nurse is a male nurse and I have mixed emotions about having a male nurse caring for my Sweetheart. I will reserve my final opinion for some later date but it could be necessary that I request a change.

Some days she is very talkative but most days she will only say a few words. Today was a talkative day and for the first time in months, she called me by my first name. I asked her how she was doing today and her response was "fine, fine, fine." It is not unusual for her to repeat the same word over and over and in most instances it has no bearing on the conversation or questions that she may have been asked. There are also times that she will be sitting at her table and start counting. She normally starts with the number one and it is seldom that her counting ever goes beyond the number eight. She does remarkably well counting in the proper sequence. In the early evening she was talking constantly but many of the words and phrases had no meaning. These are some of the things she said:

"Do you want to run out huh? It's what? We could. It's lost. He winks too. You can't have, have, have. In to. I hate to have 'em. Off any. Ver for vitch. This what. Book in there. Go out, out, out now. He's there and I do. Best you take it. Not bright. Eyes water. OK I'm giving this. Where did I have anything. You don't have it." She is cheerful and seems to enjoy just sitting, folding paper and chattering. I believe she feels at peace with the world.

Today was a very strange day. I woke her at 10:45 because it was shower day. It was very difficult to get her fully awake. When I started the waking process, it was difficult to tell if she was even breathing. I washed her face with a cold and wet cloth but that didn't seem to help. I took her outside in the bright sunlight and when I returned, she seemed to be at least partly awake. It was necessary that I feed her the bread, jam and medicine because she refused to feed herself. It was also necessary that I feed her the entire remaining breakfast meal.

After her shower she was extremely tired and laid down for a 5 hour nap. The process of trying to get her awake started all over again when I woke her. I put her into the car and took her for a drive and when I returned she was able to feed herself for the evening meal. The night meds were given without any problems but less than ½ hour later she was sleeping in her wheel chair and was wanting to get into bed. During the last 24 hours she has slept for 19 ¼ hours. I have been warned by the Hospice nurse that as the dementia progresses that she will sleep more and more.

We had visitors come during the evening hours. It was one of those rare times when things were going very, very well. She was bright, alert and very talkative. She sat at her table and spouted phrase after phrase which were punctuated with laughter. When the visitors arrived, she gave them a hearty greeting and exclaimed, "come in and take your pants off." She continued to laugh and talk during their entire visit and then bid them a warm farewell.

She has not been able to stand without assistance for well over a year. The problem is that she doesn't know that she can't stand without assistance. To guard against a fall, we have used a belt as a restraint when she was seated in the wheel chair. For several months there has been no need for a restraint because she would not attempt to stand. That came to an end today when she attempted to stand and fell. It was not a hard fall and there was no injury. The caregiver who is here two days each week immediately called the Hospice and reported the fall. The assigned Hospice male nurse came to check for injuries. The caregiver indicated that immediately following the fall that she lifted all 140 pounds from the floor and placed her into the wheel chair. The caregiver is not a large or strong person but when asked how she could possibly lift the patient, her response was the adrenalin apparently kicked in.

Along with the dementia are the problems associated with her deteriorated right hip. The pain she suffered with the bone on bone grinding was excruciating for her and was finally managed with the use of a narcotic pain patch. The patches must be changed every three days. Several days ago the hospice nurse was informed that a new pain patch prescription was needed. In the past, the new prescription has always been delivered within 2 days of the request. Three days have now passed and no new prescription. The hospice office was contacted yesterday and informed that the prescription was critically low and action must be taken or the patient would be without the required medication. If this problem isn't promptly resolved, we may be looking for a new hospice provider.

Fried trout and fried potatoes has always been one of her favorites. That was definitely not so today. She nibbled a little of the fish and a small amount of potatoes and then just refused to eat. I attempted to feed her but she just refused to eat. Finally, I gave her a small dish of ice cream and she ate it as if she was starving.

It has always been my contention that several times each day, people with dementia, may have, just for an instant, complete clarity in their thinking and understanding. That opinion was reinforced today. It was late in the afternoon and she had just risen from a nap about an hour earlier. I sidled up to her and ask her how she was doing. Her response was "I need to go to the bathroom." I hurriedly moved her into the bedroom, removed her trousers and diaper and seated her on the commode. She was correct, she did need to go to the bathroom and did.

I have bone-on-bone in my left knee and the Orthopedic Doctor has told me that my left knee should be replaced. My response was that he needed to keep me on my feet because of the caregiving responsibilities for my Sweetheart. I was putting her into bed for the night and as usual she was lifted from the wheel chair and turned 90 degrees so that she could sit on the side of the hospital bed. My left leg is the pivot leg and during the process it failed and a sharp pain was shooting from my left knee. I managed to finish the process of getting her into bed for the night and then began pondering how I could care for her if my knee became totally non-functional. The only alternative is to hire daytime in home help to perform the tasks that I could not perform or it would be necessary to place her in a care facility. Today as I am doing the caregiver tasks, they are constantly being analyzed to determine if there is a better way which will preserve my health and well-being. Those tasks where she must be lifted and then rotated 90 degrees need to be done in such a manner that my left knee doesn't become the pivot leg. That can be easily accomplished by merely backing the wheel chair to the side of the bed rather than the straight in approach that I have always used. I must become more diligent and examine all of the tasks that are performed for her care.

On her work table she has two containers that hold all of the things she works on during the day. One of the containers was an old wicker basket that has fallen into disrepair because of her constantly breaking the wicker strands. The other was a plastic basket with about 8 inch sides which were just too tall. I have been searching constantly for something better. I visited the local Walmart store and again looked for baskets without success and as I was leaving the store, I noticed a plastic serving tray. It had the low sides and was about the right size for her table. I put one in the shopping basket and continued to the check stand but then returned for another tray. I completed the purchase and as I was leaving the store, the thought struck me that maybe I should get one more and use it as a serving tray when I was feeding her at the kitchen table or when she was given some food at her table. I went back and bought another tray and they are all a big improvement over how things were done in the past. During a recent visit by a hospice nurse she noticed that I was using the serving tray when feeding my Sweetheart at the kitchen table. She commented that she had never seen that done before but it was a good idea. She went on to ask if I minded if she shared that with some of her other patients.

I just finished the monthly balancing of the check book. This task has fallen to me for the last two years but before that my Sweetheart had the task for over 54 years. Each month she balanced the check book to the penny and didn't give up until every cent was accounted for. I knew it would be done right and was never concerned about her ability to manage our funds. As I look back there are many such tasks that she assumed and of course, she did those very well also. I really didn't realize all of the things that she did until she could no longer do them and those tasks fell to me. Because of that, she was not fully appreciated for all that she has done.

I often get fully engrossed in some menial task and pay no attention to anything around me. Those times are mostly when my Sweetheart is still sleeping from the previous night or when she is napping during the day. Our home is over 43 years old and like many older homes, there are times when it creaks and groans. I will hear some sound and immediately look up to see if my Sweetheart has entered the room. For a moment, I just don't realize that she can no longer physically enter any room unless she is pushed in her wheel chair. Then I realize the impossibility of her being present and go on with what I am doing. I don't think those thoughts will ever change but that I will just keep looking up to see if she is there. I'm sure that after she is gone that I will experience those same type of thoughts and feelings.

The Hospice people told me that my Sweetheart would start sleeping more and more as the dementia progressed. I have kept a record for several months now on how much she sleeps at night and the length of her daytime naps. I reviewed those records and noted that for several months her total average sleep time was 16 hours each day. The following month the average sleep time had increased to 17 hours each day. Last month the sleep time had increased again with it averaging 18 hours each day. What will this month bring? I haven't a clue except it appears it may increase again because during the last 3 days her sleep time has been between 19 hours and 20 hours.

Our middle son who lives out of state came to visit. We picked him up at the airport when he arrived and he left the next afternoon. During his entire stay there was never any sign of recognition. The next day my Sweetheart woke early and ate a very good breakfast. When she had finished eating, she turned to the caregiver and asked "where is Darin?" Apparently the recognition was there but just never did surface until the next day following his departure. It makes me wonder what goes on in her mind that may never surface.

We are now on nurse number three. The original nurse left for work at another Hospice and she was replaced by a male nurse. I was never comfortable having a male nurse for my Sweetheart but had decided to just observe and see how things went. It was never any particular problem except two issues with her medications that were not properly or promptly handled by the male nurse. A few days ago, I received a call from the Hospice office informing me that the male nurse would be taking some personal leave and a replacement would be coming for the regular visit. The new nurse informed me on her first visit that she would be the regular nurse for the future if we were agreeable. She is a young nurse and seems very proficient in her duties and has promptly resolved any issues. She should be a "keeper" and I am much more comfortable with her coming on a regular basis.

As one gets older things just don't work as well as we think they should. Regular visits to eye doctors and regular purchase of new glasses is no guarantee that a person will be able to see very well. Today was a good example of the eyes not working well. She woke this morning with a large and very loose bowel movement. That is not an unusual occurrence so she was changed and gotten ready for her breakfast meal to be followed with a shower. I was sitting at the breakfast table and looked down at the front of my shirt, which had a white insert, and there was a large dark brown spot which was residue from changing her diaper. I immediately grabbed a spray cleaner but of course it didn't do much good. When time permitted I decided I needed to change the shirt and put it with the daily laundry. In the process, I noted another large dark brown spot on the leg of my trousers making them a candidate for the laundry also. From this experience I have concluded that I must be more careful when changing her and also, when I'm finished, stand in front of a full length mirror for a very close self- inspection.

Some of our family in the local area frequently gather and watch college football. This was one of the times when it was a late evening game. Our youngest son arrived early, greeted his Mother and sat on the couch to watch the game. My Sweetheart looked up with an angry look on her face and said "get you're a** out of here." She looked back at her magazines and toys and was immediately engrossed in rearranging things. A little later in the evening it was time for her to retire for the night. When I was preparing her for bed, the mean streak again surfaced and it was extremely difficult to get her cooperation on anything. In just a few moments the mean streak passed and she was fully cooperative in going to bed for the night. These mean streaks are not that common but it seems that they are surfacing a little more frequently as time goes by. I do have an oral dissolving medication which I can use whenever it is necessary but I'm hesitant to use it except on shower days.

Over two years ago I purchased a book that was recommended by my Sweetheart's neurologist. Apparently, after I had read the book, I completed some kind of questionnaire and recommended the book to people involved with dementia patients. I received an e-mail asking me to recommend a second book on the same subject. I had no recommendation for a second book and would have provided some narrative to that effect but that was not an option. It is my firm belief that one book is enough. That book will tell you some basic information and make some suggestions but it certainly does not provide all of the answers. Those answers won't be found in a book but will be found by trial and error on what works for you. The same thing will not work for everyone but if it works for you then use it. It is also my opinion that the authors of the books on caring for dementia patients have no direct experience. They are writing based upon hearsay. They may be highly qualified medical personnel but I don't believe they have ever walked in the moccasins of a real caregiver providing care for a loved one.

Yesterday was a banner day for bowel movements with a total of three. Needless to say, I didn't give her any more miralax. It has been a real problem trying to get her on a regular schedule. I have experimented with the amount of miralax and the frequency. I have always given her the miralax in the morning and when needed in the evening. I'm increasing the dosage to one tablespoon each day and plan to give it just before bed time. Hopefully that will give her some degree of regularity and maybe make it so she will have a daily BM in the mornings.

A neighbor and member of our church called my caregiver to see if she was interested in working at a different place. That was very upsetting to me that he would do something of that nature. I'll definitely have words with him about that and make sure he understands that his actions were inappropriate and definitely not appreciated. Our conversation will be very short, to the point and one sided. Watch your back!

Today was shower day and also the day to put color on her hair. The Hospice shower lady called and said she would come at 11:30 AM.

I timed everything accordingly and during the process of applying the hair color, she had a large BM while sitting on the shower chair. That was not a big problem but of course it was unexpected. At 11:30 AM, it was time to rinse the color from her hair and apply the shampoo – no shower lady. After the shampoo then I gave her the shower and washed her from head to toe – still no shower lady. I moved her out of the tub and started drying her and finally, 20 minutes late, the shower lady arrived. In the future I will never start anything until the shower lady is physically present. It will make more work for her but will definitely be less stressful for me and for my Sweetheart.

"Let's get out of here." "Let's go do something." "Do you know what you are doing?" "Come here and help me!" Those are some of the things that she was saying just before her bed time. Normally she doesn't talk much and when she does it is just one word here and there. It is not unusual that she only makes sounds when she is talking. No real word, just sounds that have no meaning. It was truly a pleasure to watch her and listen to her as she worked diligently at her table.

In November 2009 my sweetheart was referred to a neurologist and during the initial visit two medications were prescribed. One of the medications had some undesirable side effects so it was replaced with a similar medication in the form of a patch. In March 2013 when she was referred to Hospice, her regular doctor was asked if it was really necessary for her to continue use of the two medications. The doctor's response was that she didn't think it was necessary but to check with her neurologist. The neurologist said to discontinue one of the medications but the patch should continue to be used because "some studies have indicated that in some cases, even in the advanced stages of dementia, that discontinuance could result in behavioral problems." That response has always bothered me because there were too many "ifs" involved. In the past I have talked with the Hospice nurse about discontinuance but she was emphatic that we should not discontinue the medication. In one instance, against her wishes, I did discontinue the use and both the nurse and my caregiver believed they detected some minor behavioral problems. Three days ago I stopped applying the patch. Yesterday she was more alert than she has been in a long time and was more responsive in all areas. This morning, she woke early and ate well. Her use of eating utensils was much improved and no cleanup was necessary. When I moved her to her work table she quickly became involved with her things. At one point she picked up a small plastic picture of a young girl and said "this is a girl." I have no idea if this will continue or if it is in any way related to the discontinued use of the patch. I will be watching very closely.

Day 10 without the patch and there are no adverse effects noted. I see no reason to even consider starting use of the patch in the future. The Hospice nurse agrees.

I was moving her to the bedroom to change her diaper and lay her in the bed for the night. As we entered the hallway, for some reason, she just shot out of the chair and landed on the right side of her head on the hallway carpet. She was laying there in an awkward looking position and was crying. I tried to move her a bit and get her into a more comfortable position. The Hospice folks have said we need to immediately call them if there is a fall. I dialed their number and it just kept ringing until it ended with a busy signal. I tried the number again with the same result. Then, I called 911 and told them what had happened and that I needed assistance in getting her up and back into the wheel chair. I tried the Hospice number the 3rd time with the same results. The local fire department station is about a half mile away. They responded and were here within about 5 minutes. They provided the assistance and did a brief check for any apparent injuries and then left. In the past, I have called the Hospice after normal working hours and the telephone has been answered by an answering service. There will definitely be some discussion with them tomorrow on what is wrong with their system.

After the local fire department people arrived and she was put back into the wheel chair, they made a quick check for any apparent injuries. She was still sobbing and just wouldn't quiet down. I asked one of the firemen to hand me a piece of gum and she immediately became quite calm. I changed her diaper and put her into bed but she did not sleep immediately. During the night I awoke to a very strange silence in our bedroom. I laid and listened but could hear no sound at all. It became necessary for me to check and see if she was breathing and all was well. The whole experience was very unnerving and I laid for the longest time but sleep would not come. Finally, it became apparent that there would be no more sleep for me so I arose for the day at about 4 AM.

It is getting more of a problem for her to take the night medications. I have been giving them on a piece of bread smothered with jam but for some reason that doesn't seem to work that well at night. Tonight I took a small slice of banana bread, cut it in half and sprinkled it with the crushed medications, and then used the other half to complete a small sandwich. She just refused to even take one bite. The next effort was to put the crushed medications in a spoonful of frozen jam. She would only eat about half. The remaining jam was put on a small piece of bread which she ate with no problem. One time when I was attempting to get her to eat the medications and jam, she looked at me and said "quit bugging me!." After the last bite, I did.

It is good that Thanksgiving comes only once each year. Our Thanksgiving has just ended and it was great except it was like a zoo here at home for four days. My Sweetheart tolerated it very well and she had four days when she was very alert and talkative. She really didn't show that much recognition to anyone but she was talkative and in extremely good humor. Her shower days are on Tuesday and Friday but I was asked to change those days for Thanksgiving week to Monday and Wednesday. I agreed but did not think the situation through properly and will never agree again. The problem isn't Thanksgiving week but the time lapse between the Wednesday shower and the next regular shower on Tuesday the following week. My Sweetheart ended up getting her next shower 6 days later. I certainly understand healthcare people wanting days off but the first consideration must be for the patient. The Hospice must have the necessary staffing to provide care when needed 24/7 and anything less than that is totally unsatisfactory. I do not intend to make an issue of the situation at this time but the next time that I am approached about changing the routine, rest assured that it will be studied more thoroughly based upon what is best for the patient.

The aftermath of the Thanksgiving holiday has left myself and my Sweetheart with terrible colds. My illness is certainly more severe than hers, I think. I am constantly coughing, sneezing and have a terrible sore throat. I went to a doctor to make sure that I did not have a strep. I acquired some surgical masks to wear whenever I am around her in the event that I have a coughing spell. In her case it is impossible to tell how much discomfort she is experiencing. You can ask but she just doesn't understand and if she does understand, she doesn't know how to answer. Hopefully this will quickly pass. I need to be more careful and lessen the opportunities for her exposure whenever possible. It may be necessary when people are coming to see us to question them about colds and other illnesses and ask them not to come until those illnesses have passed.

Last night seemed to be a very bad night for her. She was coughing constantly and sounded very congested. When I try to give her something such as a cough drop, she just doesn't understand and doesn't want to take it. During the night she had several very bad coughing spells. They lasted several minutes and it was just constant coughing and sometimes gagging. In the middle of the night I tried to find a recorder so that I could record one of the spells for the Hospice nurse. After several unsuccessful tries, I finally had a recorder ready to operate. Then, of course, no coughing spells. I will keep it available during the day and hopefully if she has any coughing spell it can be captured on tape.

After a terrible weekend with no improvement, on Monday morning I sent an email to our doctor outlining our problems. In just a short time the doctor sent a reply which started with the phrase "welcome to the Thanksgiving virus." She went on to say that she has the virus and really not much can be done to speed the recovery. She did say that both of us should take daytime nyquill every four hours during the day and take nighttime nyquill before bedtime. We have followed her instructions and gained some relief. Last evening when I was preparing her drink with the nighttime medication, the measuring cup was full and I was just ready to empty it into her drink and the telephone rang which startled me. The entire bright red contents of the measuring cup was strewn on the cupboard, the backsplash and the floor. Luckily it was a tile floor and the cleanup wasn't that difficult.

Today has been a very good day. Of course, every day is a good day but some days are better than others. She is just recovering from a terrible cold and things are getting somewhere near normal. Some of the old mannerisms are starting to show up in her everyday activities. Mannerisms that she hasn't used in ages or at least I haven't noticed. Today was laced with those treasures. It is now over 21 months since a doctor certified that she would not live beyond 6 months and she was entered into the hospice program. Although sometimes have been difficult, I have never considered it a burden to care for her. I have many memories that I will cherish forever. Yes, today has been a very good day.

And thus ended the sixth day.

CHAPTER 7

The Seventh Day

T hus the heavens and the earth were finished, and all the hosts of them. And on the seventh day God ended his work which he had made; and he rested on the seventh day from all his work which he had made. And God blessed the seventh day, and sanctified it: because that in it he had rested from all his work which God created and made. Genesis 2:1-3.

Yesterday was a very, very good day. She was wide awake, alert, talking and laughing most of the day. Today was a tired day. I woke her early for her shower and she could hardly wait for a nap after the shower. She slept soundly and finally at 5 PM it was necessary to wake her. She just didn't want to wake up. I tried to feed her some stew but failed. I gave her a chocolate and she wouldn't eat it. I gave her some ice cream and she finally ate that. When it was time for her medications tonight, she was dozing in her wheel chair. She always takes her night medications on bread, the pills crushed and sprinkled on the bread and then smothered with freezer jam. Tonight she just wouldn't even take one bite. I brought a cold wash cloth to her table and washed her hands and face several times and finally she was awake enough to eat the bread, jam and medications. Bed time was at 7 PM and she was sound asleep as soon as her head laid upon the pillow.

It is the Christmas season and she doesn't even know that it is here. She just seems to live in her own world and seldom shows any signs of recognition of anything. There are times though when it seems that she recalls some of her old habits or sayings. It was not uncommon several years ago when she saw someone and they said "Hi!" that she would respond with "Lo"! Now there are times when I tell her "Hi" that she will give her old "Lo" response. I often wonder just what is going on within her mind that she just can't express but of course, I will never know.

We had our share of visitors yesterday. We had two couples drop in to visit for a short time at different times. Later in the day, one of our grandchildren and her family came to visit. It was a drive of over 350 miles to come and visit. When they arrived the two small children were not feeling that well. As the afternoon progressed, the one year old was running a temperature of over 102. After a short visit of just a few hours, they determined that they needed to return home so left to start a 350 mile drive beginning at about 8:30 PM. It was very nice of them to come and visit because we had not seen them in over 2 years. I just hope there are no adverse effects on my Sweetheart because of the children's illness.

I've been involved in surveying the various hospices in the area. I was amazed at how many there are. The purpose of my surveying was to find out what products that other hospices normally furnish, primarily the pull up diapers. The hospice that we use furnishes waterproof disposable pads for the bed, diapers that are fastened with tape, a spray to be used for cleanup after a bowel movement, and a protective salve used if a sore develops. We don't like the tape-on diapers and have never used them but have been buying our own. That ends up with a $50+ per month cost. It was interesting to note that of the six hospices that were survey, all of them furnish both pull up and tape on diapers. In addition, two of the hospices indicated that they also furnished shampoo, body wash and lotion. I was not aware that those items could be furnished and hadn't asked the question to the first 4 hospices that were surveyed. I will be having a long talk with our current hospice about what is furnished and if the results are not satisfactory then a change may be in order. I'm told the process to change from one hospice to another is a very simple process.

I received a telephone call today from the Hospice Social Worker. She said they had some kind of meeting today and were discussing the level of care for the various patients. She said she wanted to come and talk with me about the results of the meeting. They had determined that the condition of my Sweetheart had not diminished significantly and were reducing the level of care for her. When she initially entered the Hospice program, there were two visits each week from the nurse and two visits each week from the CNA whose duty was to give her a shower. Starting next week the nurse will only visit every two weeks and the CNA will only give her one shower each week. She went on to say that in about six weeks they will evaluate the patient to see if there is any deterioration that can be associated with the reduced level of care. If there is no deterioration, most likely my Sweetheart will be dropped from the Hospice program. My options are to either accept the reduced level of care or change to another Hospice. I explained to her that it will not be a fair assessment because if they reduce the showers to only one each week, then I will give the second shower myself and hire some assistance if needed. I will not under any circumstances allow my Sweetheart to go a full seven days with no shower. I have a representative from another hospice coming to visit me this week to discuss some issues and possible change.

I signed the papers to make a change to another hospice. At this point in time we are not guaranteed any specific level of care but it can't be any worse than what was proposed by the current hospice. The papers were signed at the end of the week so full transition can't take place until next week. I was instructed to call the new hospice this weekend if some kind of medical problem arises. The new hospice deals only with hospice where the old one also had home health. The old hospice had only one full time nurse and two full time CNA's whereas the new hospice has 5 full times nurses and 4 full time CNA's. I'm sure at the beginning of next week there will be considerable activity completing the transition.

Today started like most days with her sleeping until 11 AM or noon, taking morning medications and eating the morning meal. She then napped for 2-4 hours, ate the evening meal, took the night medications and is ready for bed around 7 PM. While she was awake in the afternoon, she was very alert and responded to questions and comments with real words and phrases. Most of the time she just makes sounds that have no meaning. I decided that I need to be more alert and when she says something of interest that it should be captured in the form of a note so it can be recorded in this diary. Today was a red letter day and here are some of the questions, comments and responses:

Do you want a drink? Response: I don't drink!

I love you! Response: Thank You.

Do you have a kiss for me? Response: I don't think so.

Do you want something to eat? Response: I'm working.

You're my sweetheart aren't you? Response: No I don't eat much.

A little later my caregiver and her family came by to visit and sing her some songs. They have an outstanding family choir and always sing beautifully. They sang several songs for us and sounded wonderful as always. At the end of their last song, I turned to my sweetheart and said wasn't that wonderful? Her response was "not particularly." We all had a good laugh.

It was a busy day for transitioning to the new hospice. The assigned nurse visited to gather basic information and established her schedule for two visits each week. A little later in the day the CNA called to make arrangements for the two showers each week. It appears that the showers will be on the same days and at the same times as the old hospice. Then, still later in the day the Social worker and the chaplain visited to gather basic information and they plan to visit once each month. Their visits will be separate and about 2 weeks apart. My initial reaction to the change is positive and there will be no reduction in services.

I tried the pull up diapers furnished by the new hospice. They seem much thinner and lighter than the ones that we have been using. The new diapers were used when she woke today at 11:30 and seemed quite easy to put on. She laid down for a nap at 1:30 PM and woke at 4:30 PM. When I helped her out of bed, it was noted that the bed pad was wet and her trousers were wet. I changed her immediately and the diaper did not seem that saturated but it soaked through in 5 hours. Not good. The diapers we have been using are a little bulkier but usually don't leak after 14 hours. It may be easier on the patient and the caregiver to continue using the diapers that we have been using.

I took one of the old diapers and one of the new diapers and tested them to see how much liquid they would hold without leaking. I poured an equal amount of water onto the two diapers and neither leaked. After talking with a person at the new hospice, they suggested that maybe we needed to try a smaller size to see if we could get a better fit. I am still in the testing mode but the diapers can surely be used during the day. The question still remains if they would be satisfactory for night use.

I have tried to keep my Sweetheart on some kind of schedule as nearly as possible. Night medicines are given at about 6:30 PM and she is in bed at about 7. I let her sleep in the mornings until almost noon unless it is shower day and then I must wake her a little before 11 AM. Usually about two hours after she wakes in the morning, she is ready for her afternoon nap which normally lasts upwards of two hours. If she is still napping at 5 PM then I wake her. The last few days she has changed the schedule and has been awakening around 9 AM. On those days she sometimes takes two naps during the day. I have been trying to get her back on the regular schedule but have not yet been successful.

We had a death in the family, my youngest brother. It was completely unexpected. The funeral was planned on a Friday and the caregiver agreed to come and stay starting at 9 AM on Thursday and until 7 PM the next day. The day of the funeral there was a raging snowstorm but our return was uneventful and on time. Before we left, I told my Sweetheart that my youngest brother had died. She really didn't acknowledge anything but the next day she asked the caregiver who died. She even wanted to know where I was using my name. I certainly don't like to leave her for that length of time but I know she will get care as good or better than I can give.

It is so interesting to watch her at times when she is alert and fully engaged at her table with her things. She is so meticulous in what she does and how she does it. She will carefully tear pages from her book and then very carefully fold them to make sure they are just right. She seems to eat well most of the time but it seems that more and more often I must feed her. I may feed her bite after bite and then she wants the spoon and will take a few bites on her own. Then, it seems that she forgets what to do with the spoon and lays it down. I can take the spoon and feed her a few bites and the cycle seems to start over. It is amazing that her temperament is so mild and loving. I get a great deal of personal satisfaction from caring for her.

Today was my Sweetheart's 76th birthday. My 80th birthday was four days earlier. Some of our children came for my 80th and had a flaming cake. Just prior to their visit I had decided that it was time to dispose of my Sweetheart's jewelry except for the really good stuff in our safety deposit box. We have 3 granddaughters and two daughters-in-law. I took 5 large plastic zip lock bags and a box of sandwich zip lock bags and started methodically going through the jewelry. I filled the small bags as equally as possible and placed them in the large bags. By the time I was finished each of the large bags was filled to capacity. One daughter-in-law and two grand-daughters were present for the occasion. I let each pick the bag they wanted, then the two remaining bags were given to those not present. I couldn't believe the excitement as they looked through the bags at all of the treasures. I'm sure that as the years go by, the jewelry will become more and more precious. I know that each time they wear any piece of the jewelry they will have a fond memory of where it came from and that is the way it should be. I am completely at peace with my decision and how it was done. Most importantly, I know my Sweetheart would have wanted her jewelry to be given to the family members.

My Sweetheart has been a hospice patient now for nearly 23 months. I have learned a great deal about caring for her during that time but it seems there is always more to learn. When our hospice CNA substitute gave her the shower last week, she said she had been doing that kind of work for over 27 years. After the shower was finished she was looking at some of the things that I routinely do and she was amazed that they worked so well. She immediately asked if I objected to her sharing the information with other caregivers. Of course, I had no objection. I am continually looking for different and better ways. Have you ever scrambled eggs in a microwave? I hadn't but it worked and it worked very well. I just cracked the eggs into a paper bowl, whipped them a little, nuked them for about 20 seconds, whipped them a little more, and nuked them for another 20 seconds. It was faster and the cleanup was much easier than the conventional way.

A good friend gave my Sweetheart a Costco recipe book filled with heavy shiny pages and loads of bright food pictures. She thought my Sweetheart would get a lot of enjoyment from the book. The book has been her center of attention for some time now. All of the other books and magazines have been removed from her work table. She spends a large amount of time looking at the pages, tearing the pages from the book and folding them or tearing them into small pieces. The book contains over 250 pages and the latest count shows that she is on page 98 after only about 10 days. She was diligently working on her book last evening and I was sitting next to her in a folding chair. I was constantly talking to her while she worked and suddenly she put her finger to her mouth and said sh sh sh! Needless to say, I quit talking. I'm not sure what the cost of a new book will be but regardless of cost it will be a bargain because of the joy and entertainment that she gets from the book.

A person never knows what the night will bring. She is normally put into bed at about 7 PM each night and is asleep almost instantly. I normally get into bed 2-3 hours later but check her at least hourly. She frequently kicks off the covers so it is a constant effort to check her and replace the covers. I awake quite often during the night and always check to make sure she is doing well. This past night was no different except at 3 AM she had an accident and needed to have her diaper changed. Again a little before 6 AM she had another accident and needed changed. After each change, she was back to sleep almost instantly. The accidents aren't a routine occurrence but they do happen and regardless of the time or circumstances she is changed.

Over 18 months ago my orthopedic doctor informed me that my left knee was bone-on-bone and that I needed knee replacement surgery. I told him that my Sweetheart needed to be cared for and that he needed to do what was necessary to keep me on my feet. A good knee brace was secured and it is worn every waking hour and also at night when my Sweetheart needs changed. The knee brace has been very effective. During the last month I have been experiencing some pain and wonder if time has ran out and that surgery may be the only option. Under no circumstances will my Sweetheart be placed in a nursing home so I have been pondering the best approach to continue providing in-home care. I have several different options that I am considering and I need to be prepared with the preferred option if and when the time arrives.

Another month has passed and she has reached another milestone. There have been many significant changes since she became a hospice patient but in most cases they are gradual and unnoticeable. I keep a record of her daily sleeping to include the night-time and the day-time naps. At the end of the last month her average daily sleep was exactly 19 hours each day. Eight months ago the average daily sleep was only about 16 hours each day. She eats only two meals a day but usually eats quite well. Some days she is very independent and feeds herself but then there are the days when she must be fed every bite. She continues to have a pleasing disposition and is quite pleasant to be around during her waking hours.

This has been a very unusual day. My Sweetheart awoke this morning after only 14 hours of sleep and then only napped for about one hour during the day. The past several days have been 20 hour sleep days. She has been so alert and talkative the entire day. I decided to give her a bowl of canned dark cherries for dinner. They had been canned without removing the pits. I retrieved our trusty cherry pitter and proceeded to remove the pits. When she saw the cherries she began eating them as fast as it was possible. When she finished I noticed two small pieces laying on the table. When I touched them it became apparent that they were cherry pits that the pitter had missed. After the cherries I gave her a small brownie. When she saw the brownie she exclaimed, "That's what I want!" She has continued being alert, talkative, and fully engaged at her table until it was her bed time. I'm sure that she will sleep very soundly tonight.

I'm convinced that there is no such thing as a "no call list." If there is, it is my belief that it is just a list that telemarketers ignore. Several times each day the telephone rings and the caller ID shows "private party" or some number with an unrecognizable area code. When the telephone is answered there is frequently no response from the caller or a response that it almost unrecognizable. In most instances those calls come at a time when I'm in the middle of some task for my Sweetheart and it is very difficult to get to the telephone. I know that I can just ignore the telephone and let voice mail take a message but it is not my nature to ignore telephone calls. Yesterday, a Sunday, several of those calls were received and all at very inopportune times.

Two days each week we use lots of towels. Those are the days when my Sweetheart is showered by the Hospice CNA. It is interesting to note how different CNA's have different toweling preferences. Some like large towels that are high quality and very bulky while others prefer them being not nearly as bulky. Some prefer the hand towels to do most of the drying of the patient. Two years ago when our children were inquiring about possible Christmas gifts, I told them that we needed some towels because many of ours were getting quite threadbare. They gave us one batch of towels that were very high quality and light beige in color. We received another batch of towels that were not quite the quality and were purple in color. I don't like using the high quality towel because, in my opinion it is just too bulky. It is almost impossible to dry my sweetheart's feet especially between her toes. The purple towel is not as bulky and works well for drying her feet and in-between her toes. I don't observe the rules for doing laundry very well and like to put all of the towels and washcloths into the same batch if possible. The heavy light beige towel is not a problem but the purple towel must be washed separately. I learn by doing and frequently don't realize a mistake until it is too late.

My Sweetheart has a cyst on her lower back and has had it for years. It never did cause any problems but now it is swollen and very red and ugly looking. The Hospice people won't treat it because it is not a part of that program so we went to the doctor today. At this time he is not planning on lancing it but wants to treat it with heat 3-4 times each day, continued drainage, and antibiotics. We have a prescription for 4 capsules of 500 mg each day for 10 days. That is almost insurmountable with someone who sleeps 19 hours a day and will not take pills or capsules. At this time the contents of 4 capsules is being removed and put into 16 ounces of a sweet drink. During the day we need to get 4 ounces of the drink down her at four different times. I'm sure we will be successful but it will definitely be a challenge.

The first full day of treatment for the cyst was indeed a busy day. Three heat treatments, draining and re-bandaging three times, along with giving the medications, there certainly was not much time remaining during her waking hours. I do think the day was a successful day and my Sweetheart seemed to tolerate all of the activities quite well, especially when you recognize that she was awake only 6 hours during the 24 hour period. The instructions from the doctor were 3-4 heat treatments each day. With her only awake for no more than about 6 hours, 3-4 heat treatments doesn't work very well. I believe it is necessary to just give her two heat treatments and then bandage after each treatment. A person can only do what they can do.

She slept until 11 AM this morning. After breakfast and after heat treatments, I put her into the car and we drove around the area returning some items to friends. She seemed to thoroughly enjoy her time out and about. Just before our return, we stopped at a local McDonald's for French fries and a drink. She seemed to really enjoy the fries and ate them virtually unassisted. I believed that she had an enjoyable time but when we arrived home and she was back at the table in the living room, she looked at me and said "I hate you!" I know she didn't mean it but it was still somewhat of a shocker.

The Hospice nurses have all emphasized the importance of drinking a lot of fluids. My Sweetheart never tells me when she is thirsty so many times each day she is offered something to drink. Two days ago, she would only drink a very small amount before her breakfast. When I checked the liquid, it seemed unusually cold. I placed the full glass in the microwave on high for one minute and the drink was warmed considerably but not hot. When I offered her the drink after warming, she drank most of the contents of the glass. I used the same technique the next day and today with the same results. I'm convinced that in the future the warming of her drink will make it more appetizing to her and much easier for me to increase her daily liquid intake.

I am constantly searching for different foods that she will enjoy and different ways to prepare them so they will be more palatable. She has always enjoyed eating fried chicken. My latest efforts on frying chicken was pounding chicken tenders with a cube hammer, rolling them in flour and frying. When it was time for her lunch, one half piece of chicken was cut into pieces and given her along with potatoes and gravy. She ate every bite of the chicken so I gave her a large piece just cut into strips. She enjoyed eating that chicken with her fingers and then ate half of another large piece. When dinner time arrived, I gave her another piece of chicken and she ate every bite. I'm thinking today is going to be another chicken frying day in our household.

Today is my Sweethearts anniversary. Two years ago on March 6th she was referred to the Hospice program. Things were not good two years ago. She had lost over 40 pounds, her right hip had completely deteriorated and she was always in pain. Since that time there have been many changes. She has gained back almost 30 pounds, a narcotic pain patch has been used to control the pain, and she spends her day either in a hospital bed or in a wheel chair at her table. She doesn't know anyone but of course I'm convinced that there are periodic flashes of reality where she remembers but only for short periods of time. I have become a more patient person and it is a joy to be able to provide loving care for her in our home. We do have our trials but as time goes by they are more and more insignificant. No one knows the day or the hour but of course one day the end will come and the caregiver tasks will end. I certainly was not prepared to become a full time caregiver but I will be even less prepared to no longer have the privilege of providing care.

Today is the first day of daylight savings time. I seem to always struggle with the conversion. It takes me nearly a month before the transition is complete. Although I struggle, it really has no impact on my Sweetheart. Time to her is really insignificant. She sleeps when she is tired and for a few hours each day she is wide awake. Six months ago she was sleeping an average of just over 16 hours each day. Today she spends nearly 19 hours each day sleeping which includes a daytime nap of 2-3 hours. Usually several times each month she will have a day when she sleeps in excess of 20 hours. What will the next few month bring? The Hospice nurse tells me she will sleep more and more and will start eating less and less. It is hard to believe that she could sleep more than she does now. Whatever will be will be and I just have to be ready for what comes, if that is possible.

Meals on Wheels! I'd really never given the program much thought. I decided to check out some particulars concerning the program and had a very difficult time even finding a telephone number. The person who answered the telephone asked me if I was able to drive and if my sweetheart was able to drive. I answered yes for myself and of course no for my Sweetheart. She immediately responded that I would not qualify for the program. Then, I explained to her that my Sweetheart was a Hospice patient and was bedridden, that I cared for her at home, and she must have someone caring for her 24/7. I went on to explain that of the 168 hours in each week, I was caring for her 154 hours and the other 14 hours we had another caregiver attending to her needs. She immediately told me that we both qualified for the service and that on each Monday and Wednesday, they would deliver 2 hot meals and 2 frozen meals. On Friday they would deliver 2 hot meals and 4 frozen meals for use over the weekend. It will be a week before our first meals are delivered but I'm really quite excited about that new service.

The Meals on Wheels people called on Wednesday morning and said the service would start on that day. Apparently the delivery people did not get the word because no meals came on Wednesday. Friday about noon the Meals on Wheels arrived with their first deliveries. Our first hot meal was a fish meal with vegetables and rice. It was a very tasty meal and also they sent 6 individual milk cartons, 4 individual cartons of orange juice along with bread and rolls. The weekend meals are chili/baked potato and country fried steak. I am very pleased with the initial delivery of the meals and believe that this program is going to be a great asset to us. My Sweetheart woke this morning about 11 AM and she ate some bread and jam with her medications. Other than some juice she had nothing else to eat or drink until after her shower. The Meals on Wheels people had arrived at just the right time for us to eat lunch.

I sometimes do my best thinking in the middle of the night. Last night, after a bathroom visit at 1 AM, sleep would not come. I laid for several hours pondering our lives and some of the most memorable experiences. My Sweetheart is truly a remarkable person and she has touched the lives of not only our children and grandchildren but also an untold number of other people with whom she has associated. I recall one particular instance where she was working in an office environment which supported a large number of young people doing volunteer service. One particular young lady was notified that she would be transferred to a resort area about one hundred miles to the north. She was devastated when she learned of the transfer and came to the office in tears. My Sweetheart took her aside and told her that she was being reassigned for a specific purpose. If she would go to that area, in a very short time, she would love the area, love the people, and it would be a life changing experience. Several months later, she completed the assignment and returned to her home. A short time after that, a young man from that area visited her at her home with romantic intentions. They were married and returned to that resort area to make their home where they still reside.

We've had a strange day today. Our home suffered some wind damage to the roof a short time ago and the roof is being replaced. It will be a four work day project. The day started with several workmen on the roof pounding and scraping. My Sweetheart seemed to tolerate the noise quite well. She did wake a little early but was able to nap some during the day. In the early evening a large truck arrived to deliver the new asphalt shingles and placed them on the roof. When her bedtime arrived, she seemed to be especially tired and was asleep almost instantly but a short time later she was wide awake and thrashing around the bed. I tried various things to get her to sleep but none gave results. Finally, I located some of her old sleeping pills, cut one in half and ground it. She willingly took the ground pill with a generous spoonful of frozen strawberry jam. Finally, about an hour later, she was sound asleep. It has not been necessary to use sleeping pills for several months now and hopefully the need this time was because of the turmoil with the re-roofing. It will be interesting to see what transpires during the next three workdays with people pounding and scraping on the roof.

I am always looking for better and easier ways to do things. My Sweetheart spends all of her days in either a wheelchair or hospital bed. Her clothing usually consists of a shirt, sweater, or blouse on the top with elastic wasted trousers on the bottom. It seems to be getting more and more difficult for me to lift her to a standing position and then pull up the trousers. During a normal day the trousers are often put on and removed up to four times. Our part time caregiver is a good seamstress. She has modified some of her clothing to make it easier to manage. One of my Sweetheart's dresses was black sleeveless and was made to be put on over her head and pulled down. It has been modified by cutting the dress from top to bottom in the back and installing a piece of Velcro at the top. The dress can then be slipped onto her arms over a blouse and the Velcro fastened when she is in a sitting position on the side of the bed. She is then lifted into the wheelchair. The dress can be easily removed while she is sitting in the wheelchair before she is lifted and placed into the hospital bed. The fact that some of her backside is not completely covered is immaterial when she is sitting in the wheelchair. This simple modification is a very significant labor saver for the caregiver.

Several months ago I purchased two cemetery plots close by. A headstone was also ordered from the local monument company. During the winter months the headstone could not be installed but with warmer weather the installation is now complete. We visited the cemetery to see the finished product. It couldn't be better. I know my Sweetheart didn't understand but I also know that she would be pleased with the finished product.

It seems to be a constant struggle to keep her regular. Of late, she has been given 1 heaping teaspoon of Miramax each morning. The result seems to be and early wake-up with a BM, a mid-day BM, and a bedtime BM. I'm going to try a smaller teaspoon of the Miramax and maybe give it to her mid-day. There is no magic bullet that I'm aware of but just trial and error with the hope of getting things right.

Our youngest son arrived in early afternoon to visit. A little later in the day after her naps, he went to a local drive through restaurant and picked up some fast foods for our evening meal. My sweetheart seems to really enjoy the fast foods at times. She was eating some chicken nuggets with a spicy sauce on them and really did seem to enjoy the food. As usual with spicy food, her nose started to run. I was wiping her nose constantly and she soon reached for a kleenex of her own. After she had wiped her nose I reached for the used kleenex and when she gave it to me she said "be careful, it has snot on it." I guess for that moment she was well aware of her surroundings and what was happening.

We got a call from our hospice office today. They have assigned a volunteer to us to provide assistance at various times if needed. The volunteer said she was available the following day after 5. She came and got acquainted with my Sweetheart and became familiar with our home. It was definitely an enjoyable visit for us and I believe the volunteer enjoyed her visit. I'm sure that in the future we will have more visits. The volunteer program for this hospice is a definite plus and something that the other hospice did not have.

Today was not a good day at all. My Sweetheart slept for over 20 hours counting her nap time. She was not alert at all and just seemed to be in another world. That was not really unusual. I was cooking our lunch in the oven and needed to set a timer. To be on the safe side, I usually always set two timers, one on the oven and one on the microwave. When I set the timer on the microwave, I inadvertently started it cooking with nothing inside. I never noticed my mistake until it had been cooking for nearly 12 minutes. I shut it down and opened the microwave door to help it cool down and about then everything went black. The microwave is a built-in unit and is 15 years old so my immediate thought was just to buy a new unit. I took the cabinet measurements, loaded my Sweetheart in the car and went to a very large appliance store in our area. None would fit the cabinet so the alternatives are purchase a new one and have the cabinet rebuilt or repair the old one. At this time I have opted to repair the old one but of course it is late Saturday and nothing can be done until next week. I did not realize how much the microwave was used until it wasn't available.

Caregivers never seem to have all the answers. I'm constantly learning new ways to do things. Several times each day my Sweetheart is wheeled into the bedroom and lifted out of the wheel chair and set on the side of the hospital bed. It is always a struggle during the process to sit her far enough back onto the bed to prevent her from sliding off. I have always pushed he wheel chair parallel to the bed and as close to the bed as possible. Today while moving her into the bedroom, the thought struck me that if she was angled to the side of the bed that her feet would be closer to the bed. Then, when she was lifted onto the bed it would be easier to sit her farther back onto the bed. It works!

The hospice nurse was showing me the FAST Scale – Functional Assessment Staging of Alzheimer's Disease. It was quite interesting how they evaluate patients and the various stages of their decline. The FAST Scale has 7 stages as follows:

1. Normal Adult
2. Normal Older Adult
3. Early Dementia
4. Mild Dementia
5. Moderate Dementia
6. Moderately Severe Dementia
7. Severe Dementia.

Within those 7 stages some of the items have several different identifiers. The following are more expanded identifiers for each stage:

__Stage__	__Skill Level__
1.	No difficulties, either subjectively or objectively.
2.	Complains of forgetting location of objects. Subjective word finding difficulties.
3.	Decreased job function evident to co-workers; difficulty in traveling to new locations. Decrease organizational capacity.
4.	Decreased ability to perform complex tasks, handling personal finances, difficulty marketing.
5.	Requires assistance in choosing proper clothing to wear for day, season, occasion.
6.	a. Difficulty putting clothing on properly without assistance.
	b. Unable to bathe properly, difficulty adjusting bath water temperature occasionally or increased frequency.
	c. Inability to handle mechanics of toileting (forgets to flush, doesn't wipe properly).
	d. Urinary incontinence, occasional or more frequent.

    e. Fecal incontinence, occasional or more frequent.

7.   a. Ability to speak limited to approximately a half dozen different words or fewer, in the course of an average day.

    b. Speech ability limited to the use of a single intelligible word in an average day. They may repeat the word over and over.

    c. Ambulatory ability lost (cannot walk without personal assistance).

    d. Ability to sit up without assistance lost (will fall over if there are no arm rests on the chair).

    e. Loss of the ability to smile.

My Sweetheart is definitely in Stage 7 and has been for a very long time. Still, it is a joy to be with her and watch some of her mannerisms.

We had a visit from our hospice Social Worker today. She normally visits monthly and seems to always have some particular topic that she wants to discuss. The topic today was death. In the initial packet of material that was provided was a pamphlet that outlines various things concerning the death of a patient. I re-read the material to refresh my memory and found it to be quite enlightening in some areas. Recently, I also read a small book titled "The Birth That We Call Death" by Paul H. Dunn and Richard M. Eyre. There was one particular passage that was especially meaningful:

In a beautiful blue lagoon on a clear day, a fine sailing-ship spreads its brilliant white canvas in a fresh morning breeze and sails out to the open sea. We watch her glide away magnificently through the deep blue and gradually see her grow smaller and smaller as she nears the horizon. Finally, where the sea and sky meet, she slips silently from sight, and someone near me says, "There, she is gone!" Gone where? Gone from sight—that is all. She is still as large in mast and hull and sail, still just as able to bear her load. And we can be sure that, just as we say, "There she is gone!" another says, "There, she comes!"

And thus ended the seventh day.

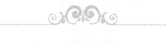

CHAPTER 8

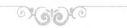

The Eighth Day

A hospice person asked if I had considered getting a Life Alert or similar system for myself. The only information I had on their system was the limited exposure from television advertisements. I was given an information paper which outlined the basics of several systems and the 2015 costs. There is a $96 installation fee and then pay $40 monthly. I was surprised at the cost. In today's environment, nearly everyone has a cell phone. I have one but only turn it on when I am away from home and someone else is staying with my Sweetheart. If my cell phone was always turned on and on my person, it would provide the same protection for me as Life Alert with no additional cost. The only difference would be that with Life Alert you just push a button and someone starts talking to you but with the cell phone you dial 911.

The hospice people have been talking with me more and more about death. They seem concerned that I will not be prepared when the time comes. I'm sure that no one is prepared but it happens anyway. I don't believe that death is very close. My Sweetheart's condition seems really quite stable. Of course there are good days and better days but that is to be expected. Each of us have those kinds of days. We have just passed the 26th month with her on hospice and I'm thinking there may be many more.

Today was Mother's Day and it was an especially good day. She woke early and then napped for just over two hours. Part of our family arrived a little after noon and I woke my Sweetheart from her nap.

She was very alert and talkative for nearly 3 hours until it was her nap time again. After she awoke from her second nap, she was very busy at her table. She has a picture on her table of our family taken last Thanksgiving. She was thoroughly engrossed in studying that picture. I'm sure that there were several people that she recognized but maybe only for a second. I will definitely remember this Mother's Day as one of the best.

Before I retired we had a saying in our office, "Don't do dumb things!" That doesn't just apply to working but really, everything in life. Today I did a dumb thing! Periodically I cut my Sweetheart's fingernails and toenails. Today was toenail day. I don't see well and my hands are very shaky. During the process of cutting the first toenail, the clippers slipped which resulted in cutting her toe. My initial reaction was just put the sock back on and the bleeding will stop. Not so! The toe of the sock was quickly saturated so I placed a dark colored hand towel under her foot. The towel was quickly soaked through and there was a large spot of blood on the light colored carpet. I wrapped it with gauze and put on a clean sock. I was telling the Hospice nurse and she offered to do all the toenail and fingernail clipping in the future. Needless to say her offer was quickly accepted.

It seems that there is always something new or unexpected happening in our lives. Today was another first. My Sweetheart received a summons for jury service in the mail. I immediately tried to call the number given in the summons but no one would answer the telephone and they wouldn't take messages. There was reference to an on-line questionnaire that each person must complete. After completion of the questionnaire, I sent an email outlining some items that could not be accommodated in the questionnaire. If a response is not received there will be no alternative but to take my Sweetheart for jury duty. I hope they have an adult diaper changing station.

It never ceases to amaze me that although my Sweetheart can't remember hardly anything, there are times when things apparently become perfectly clear. Several months ago I stumbled on the realization that she liked her drink warmed. During the process of warming her drink today, it was warmed more than normal and the glass was really quite warm. I tested the contents to make sure that it was not too warm. I offered her a drink through the straw and in the process, she touched the glass. She immediately took her hand away and said "no" and then she started blowing on the glass to help it cool. This is just another memory that I will cherish as time goes by.

For the last thirteen years at Memorial Day time there has been a gathering with my siblings. This all started the year following the death of my Mother. I just returned from the gathering and was away for two days and one night. It was an enjoyable gathering but I surely missed my Sweetheart. The return travel was started in sufficient time to permit arrival at home no later than 9 PM. Because of inclement weather the return was started a bit early and I arrived just prior to her bedtime. I immediately went to her and was greeted by a very big smile. There was no doubt in my mind that it was a smile of recognition.

I am so fortunate being able to care for my Sweetheart. Not only from the physical aspects but also because of her mild manner and sweet disposition. When she is laid in bed, she is asleep almost instantly and nearly always sleeps the entire night. When she does wake there are no signs of agitation and she never makes any loud noises. She will lay quietly just looking at the ceiling and sometimes muttering to herself. When she is sleeping during the day I'm constantly going to the bedroom to make sure all is well.

It was a sad day today! My microwave died. It was a built in unit and when it needed repair I was willing to pay whatever was needed to get it repaired. The final repair cost was just short of $600. It never did work properly and the repair people returned several times and the last visit they said that there was nothing more that could be done. They went on to say, use it until it dies. I started looking for something that would fit into the built-in slot and sit on a shelf. I finally found a unit on the internet and it will arrive within the next two days. Not bad, I paid nearly $600 to fix the old one and the new unit costs $140. At least I will have a microwave.

I'm always amazed at what my Sweetheart can remember at times. After her shower when she is dried, clothing is put on her top. She needs no coaxing but immediately reaches for the bottom of the garment and pulls it down, front and back. She doesn't eat well with a fork. A spoon is the preferred eating utensil but there are times when she turns the spoon upside down and tries to eat. She will work diligently to get food to cling to the rounded part of the spoon. She may need to be prompted to turn the spoon over but there are times when she turns it without prompting.

It was late in the afternoon and she was sitting at her table. She did not seem alert at all and was not much interested in anything. I sat down in the folding chair beside her and tried to talk with her but nothing seemed to register. Then she took my hand, squeezed it and put it to her mouth and kissed it. In just a moment, she repeated the squeezing and kissing, then she smiled. Those are the moments that make lasting memories.

Some things are predictable but most things are not with regard to dementia. The morning wake-up time varies from 7:30 AM to 1 PM and there is no way that a person can plan. Some days she will feed herself every bite but other days she must be fed. It is interesting to watch as she feeds herself because invariably sometime during the meal she will turn the spoon upside down and try diligently to scoop food. There are days when she is sitting at her table and after a short period of time the floor and the table will be littered with small pieces of paper that she has torn from a clothing catalog. Other days, she busies herself at the table but never touches one of the catalogs. Frequently when she is engrossed in her efforts at the table, I will call her name to get her attention. Most recently her name was repeated several times with no visible response but finally, without even looking up, she responded "I can hear!"

Our regular hospice nurse shares the same wedding anniversary date with us. She is taking that week off work and has been working diligently to get all medications ordered and delivered before her departure. She placed the order on a Tuesday and said they should be delivered on Wednesday – not so! Thursday came and went with no delivery. Friday morning I alerted the hospice that we still did not have the required medications. After some telephone calls, I was assured that they would be delivered that afternoon. I learned long ago that when medications are delivered that they should be closely examined before signing. Today, the narcotic pain patch that was delivered was not the proper patch and was supposedly the reason for the delay. However, the patch was acceptable but just did not adhere to the patient in the desired manner. My Sweetheart has been taking a certain generic medication for several years but the delivery today was for a completely different medication. I questioned the delivery man who, of course, had no answers, and called the pharmacy who could not satisfactorily explain. I then called the hospice and reported the problem and refused to sign for that medication. Some three hours later, the proper medication was delivered. I'm not exactly sure who is directly responsible for the problem but I intend to find out.

Yesterday my Sweetheart was very alert during all of her waking hours. She sat at her table, working diligently and always had an answer of some type when she was addressed. She was responding with sentences or phrases most of the time. Today was just the opposite. She hardly ever responded when addressed and just was not alert at all. It will be interesting to see what tomorrow brings. I learned long ago to expect the unexpected whatever that may be.

The meals on wheels are delivered in a tinfoil container so if they are heated in the container, it must be done in a conventional oven. That seemed to work well but of course it is rather time consuming when compared to a microwave. Lately, I have been removing the meal from the tinfoil container and placing it in a microwaveable bowl. Today when it came out of the microwave, the bowl was quite warm. I stirred the contents and tasted the food to make sure it wasn't too hot. When I gave her the food, she touched the bowl and noticed that it was quite warm. She took some food and touched it lightly with her tongue then touched it with her tongue again. Apparently she decided that it was not too warm to eat and began eating. I know that sometimes her mind definitely does work.

Our regular hospice nurse is taking vacation this week so we were visited today by a substitute nurse. The visit went extremely well and just as he was leaving he remarked the outside rings on the wheels of the wheel chair could be easily removed making it much more maneuverable. The outside rings are installed for patients who have some degree of mobility by moving themselves around. I had never considered removing the outside rings but as soon as the nurse had departed, off came the outside rings. Yes, the wheel chair is much more maneuverable in our home. It has the same effect as widening each doorway by 4 inches.

My Sweetheart just hasn't been sleeping that well since the start of daylight savings time. The master bedroom in our home has 4 large ceiling to floor windows. It seems that the morning sun streams through making the bedroom extremely bright. Today a dark colored king sized flat sheet was pinned in such a manner that it covered the in-place draperies and darkened the room considerably. This should improve her sleeping in the early morning and is a definite improvement for her daytime naps.

At least weekly I am asked how well is she sleeping and how much does she sleep. Over a year ago, I decided that if I was going to give accurate information that some kind of record needed to be maintained. I developed a one page monthly record where her night-time sleep and her daytime sleep could be recorded on a daily basis from that information it was easy to determine her average daily sleeping time. The figure below shows a copy of the actual record for one month.

MONTH	JUN	NIGHT				NAP			
Date	In Bed	Awake	Hours		In Bed	Awake	Hours		Total Hours
1	6:45	9:15	14 1/2		11:30	4:00	4 1/2		19
2	6:45	~~11:15~~ 10:45	~~16 1/2~~	BM	2:45	5:30	2 3/4		20 3/4
3	7:15	11:00	16 1/4		1:30	3:30	2		18 1/4
4	6:45	7:45	13	BM	12:30 9:45-11:30	3:00	2 1/2 1 3/4		17 1/4
5	6:30	11:30	17		1:15	3:45	2 1/2		19 1/2
6	6:45	10:00	15 1/4		11:15	2:15	3		18 1/4
7	6:30	7:45	13 1/4	BM	3:00 9:00	4:45 1:15	4 1/4		18 1/2
8	7:00	11:00	16		12:45	3:45	3		19
9	7:00	10:00	15		12:30	3:00	2 1/2		17 1/2
10	7:00	7:30	12 1/2	BM	9:30-11:30	1:45-3:30	3 3/4		16 1/4
11	7:00	9:30	14 1/2	BM	12:00	3:00	3		17 1/2
12	7:00	9:30	14 1/2	BM	12:00	3:00	3		17 1/2
13	6:45	7:45	13	BM	2:00 9:15	3:15 11:15	1 1/4 2		16 1/4
14	7:00	11:00	16		12:15	3:15	3		19
wt 138 15	6:45	9:15	14 1/2	BM	11:45	3:15	3 1/2		18
16	6:45	8:15	13 1/2	BM	1:30 10:00	3:45 12:00	2 1/4 2		17 3/4
17	6:45	11:00	16 1/4		2:00	4:00	2		18 1/4
18	6:45	8:30	13 3/4	BM	10:00-11:30	1:30-2:00	2		15 3/4
19	6:30	8:30	14	BM	10:30	1:15	2 3/4		16 3/4
20	6:45	11:00	16 1/4		12:30	3:45	3 1/4		19 1/2
21	6:45	9:15	14 1/2	BM	3:00 10:30	4:00 1:30	1 3		18 1/2
22	6:45	8:45	14		~~12:45~~	No NAP			14
23	6:45	9:45	15	BM	12:45	4:15	3 1/2		18 1/2
24	7:00	10:30	15 1/2	BM	12:00	3:30	3 1/2		19
25	7:00	9:15	14 1/4	BM	11:00	1:45	2 3/4		17
26	6:45	11:30	16 3/4		1:00	4:15	3 1/4		20
27	7:00	10:45	15 3/4		12:30	3:30	3		18 3/4
28	6:45	9:45	15	BM	11:45	2:45	3		18
29	6:45	10:45	16	BM	12:00	4:00	4		20
wt 134 30	6:45	11:00	16 1/4		12:30	4:00	3 1/2		19 3/4
~~31~~					18.1				
				30	544 30		18.1 Average		
Totals					244 240				

40 30 10

181 + 3 1/4 = 184 1/4

172 + 4 1/4 = 176 1/4

181 + 2 1/2 = 183 1/2

183 1/2
176 1/4
184 1/4
543
+ 1
544

After I had kept a similar record for a few months, I decided that it would be more meaningful if the monthly results were put on a line graph. The next figure shows the actual results since the records have been maintained.

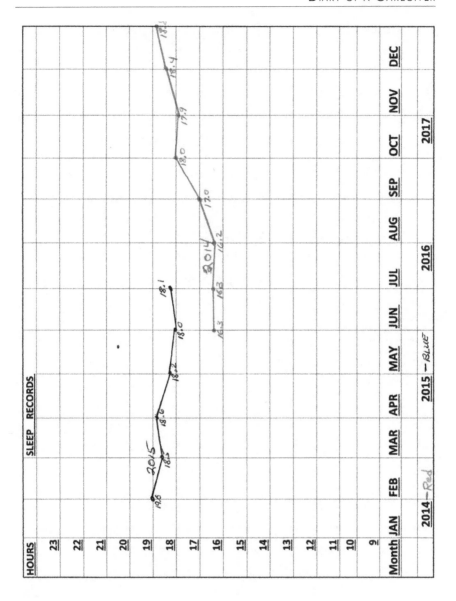

There certainly may be a better way but this works for me. Now when I am asked the question of how well or how much she is sleeping, I have a good answer at my fingertips and I can show the increased average daily sleep time for many months.

We are in the middle of a very hot spell. Normally we have less than a dozen days of triple digit temperatures each year. With the days we have already had that were triple digit and those forecasted in the next two weeks, we may be close to 20 days and we are not even into the hot months. We don't venture outside anymore than is necessary. If it is necessary to put her into the car and run an errand, leaving her in the car alone is not an option.

I use a lot of paper products. I recently ordered a large supply of plates, saucers, and small bowls from the internet. In the past, in most instances her food was put on a paper plate. It worked well but there were times when she had some difficulty getting the food onto her eating utinsel. Over time I have determined that she does much better eating her meals with a spoon. Also, I have determined that it is much easier for her to eat when her food is put into a cereal bowl rather than placing it on a paper plate. She seems to be able to manage getting the food onto the spoon and into her mouth much better. There may be cases where she will have a meat, and two vegetables in the same dish but the mixing of them doesn't appear to be a problem. When the same items were on a plate, they ultimately ended up being mixed together during the eating process. She just does better with the food in a bowl.

Today I need to go grocery shopping. Someone from our church is coming at 1 PM to stay with her while I'm out and about. My plan was to let her sleep until 11 AM, feed her the breakfast meal, and lay her down for a nap at 12:30. I could safely complete my shopping and errands in plenty of time before she would awaken. The plan didn't work. She woke this morning at 9:00 AM with a bowel movement, ate and then laid down for a nap at 11:00. I'm not sure if she will stay asleep while doing the shopping. We will see and as always, adjust as necessary.

I enjoy fresh dark cherries and my Sweetheart always enjoyed them also. Today at the grocery store I bought a one pound bag with the intent of just eating them fresh. I remember last year when I bought cherries they were pitted and then some were given to my Sweetheart. Well, cherry pitters work well but are definitely not foolproof. After she had eaten the cherries, I noticed two small red blobs and they were cherry pits that she had spit out. I decided today to give her one cherry with the pit inside and see if she would spit out the pit. Bad decision, she wouldn't spit out the pit but continued to try and crush it between her teeth. I coaxed and pleaded to no avail. What happened to the cherry pit? It most surely was swallowed because in didn't come out of her mouth. No more fresh cherries unless the pits are removed.

I needed to make a grocery run and asked my caregiver if there was something that she thought I needed to buy. She mentioned that she was eating some yogurt and offered some to my Sweetheart and that she seemed to enjoy it. She was never a big yogurt fan but when she did eat some, she seemed to prefer the key lime flavor. I bought several containers of key lime and two containers of peach. The contents of a container were removed and put into a cereal bowl and she seemed to really enjoy it. She had eaten the key lime several times so I gave her some peach yogurt. She took one bite and refused to eat any more. She likes peaches so I cut up a half peach into small pieces and mixed it with the yogurt. It didn't help. One bite and not another. She still knows what she likes.

My hands shake! I've had that problem for years and it seems to have gotten progressively worse. When I was still working, I would frequently play golf with friends. They often said that my hands shake so bad that I could hardly keep score but when I'm standing over a putt worth $5 that I'm steady as a rock. I've tried various medications over the years but none seemed to help so I just live with it. People make adjustments in how they do things to compensate and it frequently helps. I'm right handed and it seems that my right hand shakes more than the left but maybe that is because it is more noticeable. When I'm pouring a drink my elbow is often braced against my body which sometimes minimizes the shakes. Some days there is a real problem when feeding my Sweetheart. Often I will do the feeding with my left hand or at times it is necessary to use both hands. The shakes really don't pose a major problem but just another thing to contend with when caregiving.

Today was the day of the big sleep. My Sweetheart was put into the hospital bed last evening at 6:45. Today she was still sleeping at 1:15 PM so I woke her for some lunch and her medications. One hour later she was napping in her wheel chair so back into bed. She was still sleeping at 5 PM so I woke her again. When she is in bed, she lays on her back and just doesn't move at all. She is laying in the same position when she awakens as when she was laid down for sleep. Over 21 hours of sleep for today is almost unreal.

I was notified today that some items that were ordered for me have now arrived and need to be picked up. The location was some sixty miles to the West. I put my Sweetheart in the car, fastened her seatbelt and we started the drive. All went well until part way through the return and then she became quite upset. Trying to console her and driving at the same time became quite difficult. She finally calmed and the remainder of the trip was uneventful. She was very glad to be back home and in familiar surroundings. The two + hour drive was just too long.

I woke her this morning at 10:45 AM because it is her shower day. The hospice CNA comes at 11:30 AM and about 45 minutes is needed to change her diaper, give her the morning medications and breakfast. It was almost impossible to get her fully awake. Finally I kept washing her face with a wet wash cloth. When it was medication time, they are given on a small jam sandwich, she would hardly eat but finally ate the entire sandwich. Her preferred cereal is Honey Smacks and she dearly loves them. Today, it was a struggle from the first bite to get her to eat. There was also some difficulty yesterday.

Have you ever noticed that people who are not involved in caregiving always have lots of suggestions on how it should be done. Sometimes, it results in actual criticism of nearly everything. They mean well and on rare occasions they may have suggestions with some merit. There is no school solution and I'm sure that every patient is different. The best way for one patient may not work at all for another. It is a constant effort of trial and error and when we find what we consider the best way, it may not be the best way for next week or next month. We just have to do the best that we can.

I have fabricated something so I can weigh my Sweetheart when she is sitting in her wheel chair. I place a set of bathroom scales on the tile floor, put the framework in place, and rolled the wheel chair to the balance point and then locked the wheels. I can then read the weight shown on the scales, subtract 52 pounds and that is her body weight. I monitor her weight several times each month and try to keep her weight somewhat constant. I recently re-done the framework using 2 fence boards that were 6 feet tall by 5 ½ inches wide. Below is a picture of the finished product. It works!

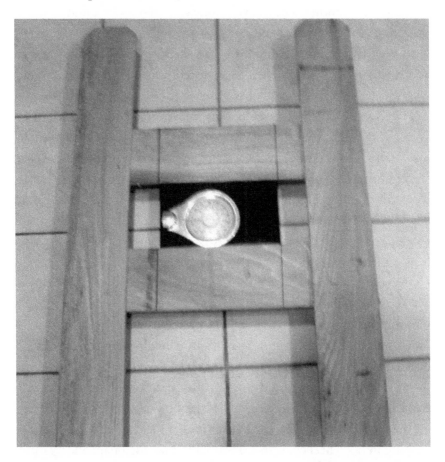

Most days, my Sweetheart doesn't talk that much but then some days she talks constantly. I sidled up to her today, one of her talkative days, and asked if she would give me a kiss. She immediately had a response, "Someday." Life is good.

The hospice furnishes a waterproof absorbent pad to use on the hospital bed or to cover the pad in the wheel chair. The waterproof pad is 30 X 30 inches and is a definite asset when it comes to keeping the bedding clean. I place one of the pads on the far side of the hospital bed and it covers about 2/3 of the width of the bed. Then, I place another pad on the near side of the bed and it covers about 2/3 of the width.

When my Sweetheart has an accident, the diaper is removed and she is partially cleaned and then one of the soiled pads is removed and replaced with another. The final cleaning can then be done and by using the two pad method the bedding is seldom soiled.

Recently, the hospice order for the absorbent pads did not arrive and their supply was completely exhausted. On a Friday morning my Sweetheart had an especially messy bowel movement and several pads were needed. After final cleanup, only one unused pad remained. The hospice was contacted and could not help. When I had changed to a different hospice seven months ago, the remaining supplies from the old hospice had been moved to a closet for a backup stock. It was fortunate that the backup supplies were available because during that day she had two more instances where pads were needed. The hospice order finally arrived over seven days late and my backup stocks have been replenished.

Keeping her bowel movements regular is always a concern. I rely on Miralax and have been giving her two teaspoons when she arose each morning. The last seven days she has awoke early with a large bowel movement and then never seems to get enough sleep for the day. I decided that the Miralax dosage should be delayed until the afternoon so her morning sleep would not be interrupted. She slept very well last night and was still sleeping at 1 PM. She was awakened, given her morning medications and her mid-day meal. Within an hour she was sleeping in her wheel chair so she was laid down for a nap. She was still napping at 5:15 PM. She was awakened, given an evening meal and her night medications and in less than 2 hours she was tired and ready for bed. Her total sleep time today was 21 ¾ hours. There is hardly enough time to feed her 2 meals and give medications.

A few months ago we discontinued using a mild sleep aid medication that had been prescribed. Initially it appeared that there was some difficulty getting to sleep so a very low dose of melatonin was given with her night medications. I recently purchased some 1mg melatonin tablets of a different brand and gave her ½ of a tablet. She seemed very restless during the night and was wide awake at 6 AM the next morning. I changed her diaper and put her back into bed. She was asleep immediately but then seemed very restless. I'm not sure if the cause is the different brand of melatonin or just a periodic natural occurrence but I'm sure that time will tell.

We have a master bath in our home plus a main bathroom on the ground floor. In the past the towel rod in the main bathroom always had decorative towels displayed. They have long since been removed and only one everyday hand towel is displayed. It seems that each time someone enters the bathroom the hand towel, for some reason, falls to the floor. During my Sweethearts shower, the CNA commented that the falling towel problem could be solved by putting a few small dots of regular calk along the towel rod. It worked!

Today was one of those rare days that I will always fondly remember. My Sweetheart woke earlier, napped a little less than usual but was so alert and talkative that it was almost unbelievable. She sat at her table and was very busy with her toys and magazines. Each time anyone approached her they were greeted with a very large smile and she was talking constantly. She was like the ever ready battery bunny and just didn't slow down. After she took her night medications the alertness continued until it was her bedtime. Here again, when her head hit the pillow she was sound asleep.

The monthly medications were delivered today. I always check the medications to make sure they are the ones prescribed. Not so today. One of prescribed medications is the generic for Lexapro but the delivery was the generic for Celexa. I don't know who messed up but for sure someone did.

It was early in the morning and for some reason she was awake and seemed quite agitated. My initial thought was that she had a bowel movement and needed changed. Not so but her diaper was removed and she was sat on the commode. Immediately she had a large bowel movement in the commode. In my opinion, another example of her thinking clearly for just a few moments. Her agitation was apparently her way of showing that she needed to use the commode.

Monday and Thursdays at 11:30 AM are designated shower days and time for my Sweetheart. Last Monday the regular CNA was off so a substitute was assigned but the time was unknown. Finally at 3:30

PM the substitute CNA arrived and my Sweetheart was in the midst of a deep sleep. Today, Thursday, the CNA called at 8:45 AM and asked if she could come at 9:30 AM. She was told that my Sweetheart was sleeping soundly and I didn't want to awaken her. My caregiver came at 9 AM and at 9:45 AM the CNA called again and wanted to come early. She was told that my Sweetheart was still sleeping soundly. The CNA called again at 10:30 AM and said she would be coming later in the day. She finally arrived at 2:30 PM and of course, my Sweetheart was in the middle of another deep sleep. There will be some discussions with the CNA at my next opportunity. I certainly have no problem with her coming early when my Sweetheart awakens early but to come 3 hours later than our designated time is totally unacceptable. She will be reminded that the welfare of the patient must come first.

Caring for someone who is bedridden definitely is challenging. It can be difficult to do the required lifting to and from the wheel chair, to and from the bed, and to and from the commode. One of the benefits is that a person doesn't have to contend with the problems associated with wandering. I frequently talk with people who are caring for a loved one who wanders and can only imagine some of the problems that they face. I also talk with people caring for a loved one who is combative. I am truly blessed because wandering and combative problems are not an issue.

My Sweetheart's day is spent in one of three places: in the hospital bed sleeping, at the table in the kitchen eating her meals or at her table in the living room. She seems very stable and I'm convinced that a significant contributing factor to her stability is her table. It is loaded with things that she enjoys handling, tearing, folding or just playing with. When I've visited care facilities I've noticed the majority of the patients just sit on chairs or at tables and stare into space. That is not so with my Sweetheart. Her hands are busy doing something and she seemed totally engrossed in her activities. I have a box of items that have been on the table at times and will be rotated back when she has lost interest in other items. Her table is positioned directly in front of the TV so she can just look up and see the picture. She seldom watches the

TV unless it catches her interest. This is a picture of her table at the end of the day right after she was laid down to sleep for the night.

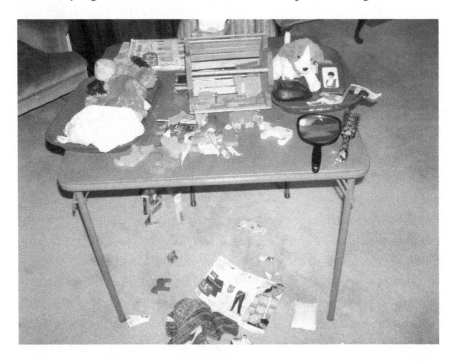

The hospital bed has side rails at both the head and the foot. When my Sweetheart is sleeping, the side rails are always raised to prevent a fall. During her time sleeping, she never seems to move. She doesn't toss or turn and the sheets and blankets stay in the same place during her entire sleep. This morning as she lay sleeping, I had a strange feeling that the end may be getting near. As that thought crept into my mind, my immediate reaction was that I'm certainly not prepared. I don't believe a person is ever prepared.

Meals on Wheels has been a very good program for us and have always been delivered within about a one hour window. Today, that was not the case. At 1:30 PM, no meals had been delivered so I called the office of the coordinator. Of course no one answered the telephone but in addition to the normal message, a cell telephone number was provided for immediate assistance. That number was called and of course no answer but I did leave a message. At 3 PM there was still no response so I called again and this time a real person answered. They had no explanation for why meals were not delivered but assured me that they would call back. About 20 minutes later they called and said they had no idea why meals weren't delivered but someone would be delivering them by 5 PM. At 6 PM still no meals but finally they arrived about 6:30 PM.

We were notified of a change to the Meals on Wheels delivery. In the past we received a hot meal and a frozen meal on Mondays & Wednesdays with a hot meal and two frozen meals on Fridays. The meal delivery schedule has now changed to a hot meal and six frozen meals on Tuesdays. This new schedule should work just as well as the old schedule.

My Sweetheart never ceases to amaze me. She doesn't know me but at times there are short flashes of recognition. She can't speak and doesn't understand when she is spoken to. She has difficulty feeding herself but when she is fed something and a small part of the food is hanging outside her mouth, she never hesitates on manipulating her mouth and lips to get the food into her mouth. I took her for a short ride today in the car. When she is lifted out of the wheel chair, turned and sat on the edge of the seat, she immediately knows that she must slide back in the seat and raise her legs so she can be turned and properly seated. We were riding and turned the car into the setting sun, she immediately reached for the sun visor and pulled it down to shade her eyes. When we arrived home and pulled into the garage she started trying to remove her seat belt. I unhooked the seatbelt and opened her door, she immediately tried to raise her legs and turn in the seat. It was not a long ride but I'm sure that she thoroughly enjoyed the ride and the time out of our home.

Her medications for both morning and night are ground and capsules are emptied. The morning medications are given in a jam sandwich made with one slice of bread. The night medications are given on 1/2 slice of bread smothered with jam. I live in fear of the day when she will no longer take the medications. Tonight I thought that day had arrived. I pleaded and coaxed for nearly 15 minutes until she finally took the first bite and then she eagerly ate all that remained.

Today is my Sweetheart's anniversary. She has now been a hospice patient for thirty two months. There have been a lot of changes since she entered the program but for the last several months she has been quite stable. Of course there have been some days when she just did not do well but those are in a minority. I have so many memories while caring for her and consider it to be a privilege.

A few days ago I visited my friendly dermatologist. As usual, he froze several suspicious areas and took one biopsy. The results indicated an aggressive skin cancer on the left side of my face. Today was removal day and I am now sporting a large bandage for the next week. Needless to say, it is very tender to the touch and should not be bumped. Little did I realize how difficult it is to guard it when lifting and caring for my Sweetheart. We have an outstanding caregiver who helps me two days each week but she has a family of her own and there definitely will be times that her family requirements will supersede my requirements. I need a backup plan! I called a local Personal Care Service (PCS) agency today and have an appointment in a few days for them to explain their program, rates and requirements. They will make an on-site assessment of our needs. I need to have all the arrangements made and all paperwork completed so when the time comes one telephone call will activate the plan.

I met with the Personal Care Service person today and she gave me a packet to read with some forms to be completed. She indicated that there appears to be a shortage of caregiving personnel and there is no guarantee that if I have a need that it can be filled. While she was here we talked about the demanding caregiving requirements. I showed her my shower transfer bench with the swivel seat and the seat that slides the patient from outside the tub. She indicated that she had been in the health care business for over 15 years but never had she seen anything of that nature. She told me of a current patient who may have to be placed in a care facility because of the great difficulty that they have getting her into and out of the tub for her showers. She took pictures and a video so she could show it to the family members who have a need. This is a picture of the transfer bench.

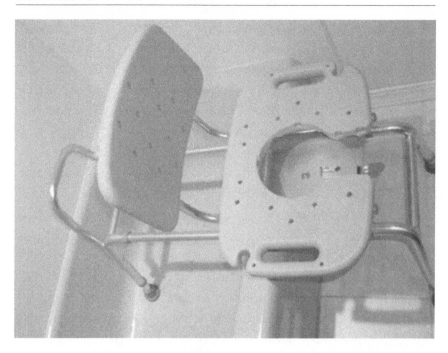

This was a very strange day today. My Sweetheart woke quite early with a very large bowel movement and was not interested in going back to sleep. Two hours later it was back in bed but her normal nap was only about half as long as usual. A little later in the day she was laid down for another nap but only stayed about one hour. It has been one of those days were she was very alert and talkative. She just didn't seem to get tired and was constantly working at her table on something. I'm sure that tomorrow will be vastly different and will be a sleep catch up day for her.

Today was a very routine day and my Sweetheart was not very alert. Along towards evening she was sitting at her table and was mostly staring into space. I asked her some simple question. She immediately straightened up, spread her arms apart and exclaimed "wheeeee." I responded with a question of how she was doing. She immediately said "don't ask me." The responses and mannerisms were reminiscent of days gone by. I never know what to expect or when to expect it but that keeps life interesting.

I always heat my Sweetheart's drink in the microwave until it is luke warm. She drinks with a straw but somedays it seems that she doesn't know how to drink. I keep offering the straw to her but after several times it is often necessary to "prime the pump" with a drink from the glass. In those instances after she has a small drink from the glass, the straw is offered and she drinks without any further problems.

Daylight savings time ended this morning at 2 AM. It always seems to take me a long time to adjust to the one hour change. Last evening all of our clocks were set back one hour which should mean that I can sleep an hour longer. For some strange reason, I awoke one hour earlier than my usual 5 AM which showed on the reset clock as 3 AM. I tried and tried to get back to sleep but finally just gave up. I'm wondering if this change will have any effect on my Sweetheart.

I always wonder what she is thinking, what she is remembering and what she senses. Of course there is no way of knowing but I still wonder. I always look forward to my off days and normally leave at 9 AM and return by 4 PM. Seldom is she awake before 9 AM except on my off days she seems to awaken earlier than normal. In fact, on most of my off days she awakens early enough that I can get her out of bed and at least partially feed her. I'm convinced that some way she senses that I will be leaving and awakens before my departure.

She woke a little early this morning and ate a good breakfast and was soon ready for a 4 hour nap. While she was still sleeping visitors came to see her. I always tell people that if they come between 4 and 6 PM, she will always be awake. Naturally they were a little early but she awakened in time for them to see her. She was not alert at all but just sat and stared into space. After the visitors departed she ate a good dinner meal and then was alert and very busy the rest of the evening. It is impossible to know what to expect from hour to hour or day to day.

A few days ago I was sitting next to my Sweetheart and her response to a question was "I don't know what to do." That response has been on my mind for several days as that same response was given sometime in the past. After much pondering, I recalled the circumstances for the response. Over three years ago my Sweetheart and I were being interviewed by our church officials. At the time of the last interview I suggested to the official that we be interviewed together. His response was that they didn't like to do that but wanted to interview us separately.

After my insistence, he finally reluctantly agreed to a joint interview. We entered the interview room and he turned to my Sweetheart and asked that she offer a short prayer prior to the beginning of the interview. She sat for a minute and finally responded "I don't know what to do." During her lifetime she had probably offered thousands of prayers without hesitation but it was just no longer possible.

A good friend sent an email with this internet link to a video that he suggested I view. It was a video of an older gentlemen with severe tremors providing loving care to his Sweetheart who was severely incapacitated. It was a short and very touching video it made me very sad. I thought of my own situation and how blessed that I am to be in the circumstances that I enjoy. My response to my friend was that I plan to keep the link to the video and view it again if I think I am having a bad day.

It was a strange day today. Because of some of my health issues I needed to be at the Doctor's office at 8 AM. My Caregiver had agreed to come to work early at 7:45 AM rather than the normal 9 AM. At 7:30 this morning my Sweetheart was wide awake. Her night time sleep was just over 12 hours which was an all-time low. I was sure it would be a two nap day and it was. While she was sitting at her table between naps, she picked up her hand held mirror, looked into it and said "I Love You!" After her last nap ended she was really quite alert. I gave her a small dish with mixed nuts and skittles. First she carefully ate the cashews then the skittles and finally the remaining nuts. It was so interesting watching her and how intently she focused on her task. Finally, it was medication time for her at 6:15 PM and in just a few minutes she was overtaken by exhaustion. I laid her in the hospital bed and she was quickly sound asleep.

Our youngest son who lives in the area came to visit this past weekend. He was sitting at the work table by his Mother and put his golf cap on her head. She really seemed to like having a cap on and resisted when he attempted to retrieve it. One of my golf caps was adjusted to fit her head and since that time she frequently wears the cap during most of her waking hours. She never attempts to remove it and is perfectly content working at her table. During the last few days while she has been wearing the cap, she has been extremely alert and talkative. She talks mostly in short sentences and frequently answers questions without hesitation. It is unbelievable that wearing a cap would have such a positive impact but at this time there is no other explanation.

The holiday season has always been a special time of year. Thanksgiving time seems to be the time for our family gatherings and this year was no different. My Sweetheart tolerated things well and the confusion didn't seem to upset her at all. I woke her early so we could take family photos then she napped. I woke her from the nap for Thanksgiving dinner and a little later she napped. Then she woke herself towards the evening hour. As she was given some of her favorite food from her own recipes, you could see a sparkle of enjoyment in her eyes. I'm sure that she had some recollection of bygone days.

We've had over two days of vigorous activities in our home which is normally very quiet and peaceful. My Sweetheart seemed to enjoy every minute. She is normally very stingy giving out kisses but on the final day as our family members were leaving to return to their homes, as each bid their final goodbyes, she gave each a big kiss. She didn't know anyone's name but she knew that each was a special family member.

And thus ended the eighth day.

CHAPTER 9

The Ninth Day

Our local newspaper today had a lengthy article titled "Caregivers Feel Pain, Relief, Guilt." The article was addressing an Alzheimer's patient and was really quite well written. It outlined some of the problems associated with caregiving but I am still confused about the title of the article. I just can't associate any of my caregiving activities with pain, relief or guilt. Maybe I'm doing something all wrong.

I am a little worried today. Last evening, over an hour before her normal time to take the night meds, she was sleeping in her wheel chair. Her meds were hurriedly prepared and after several attempts it was necessary to wash her face several times with a cold wash cloth to get her fully awake. Then, she took her meds with no problems and was put into bed a full hour before her normal bedtime. She was still sleeping soundly today at 1 PM. I woke her, gave her the morning meds and fed her the normal morning meal. She ate well at first but a little later it required significant effort to get her to finish her meal. She was moved to her table and at 2 PM she was again sleeping soundly in her wheel chair. She was put into bed for a nap and today ended up being a sleep day of over 22 hours.

My Sweetheart had some favorite foods that she really enjoyed. I was at a local grocery store and noted the smell of freshly baked apple fritters, one of her favorites. One was brought home and cut into small pieces. At the first bite it was obvious that she remembered the taste.

She also enjoyed an orange jello, cheese and pineapple salad. She was given a small dish of the salad and again, it was easy to tell that she remembered the taste.

It was a routine diaper change but in the process my Sweetheart grabbed the pads that protect the bedding. In an effort to free the pads from her grasp and to finish pulling up the diaper, her good leg started to give away. I attempted to seat her back onto the bed but she was too close to the edge and slipped to the floor. I knew from past experience that it was not wise for an 80 year old to try to lift her back onto the bed. She was positioned in a sitting position on the floor with her back against the hospital bed and with a bed pillow behind her back. The hospice was called and in just a few minutes help arrived and she was re-seated on the bed. It was fortunate that there was no injury.

Today was her shower day and when the shower lady called about 9:30, my Sweetheart was still sleeping. I told the shower lady that I would wake her and give her the morning medications before her shower. She just wouldn't awaken. Her face was bathed with a cold wash cloth but still she wouldn't drink or eat anything. Finally, in desperation, some music was put on the television, the volume turned up, and I danced with her in the wheel chair. In a very short time she was wide awake, ate the sandwich with her medications and was ready for her shower. The next time there is difficulty in getting her wide awake, the music and the dancing may be the best choice.

She was sitting at the table and had just finished eating her breakfast. I was in the process of washing the dishes and inadvertently bumped a pan against the side of the sink making a loud noise. My Sweetheart's immediate response was "don't break it." A little later I sneezed a very loud sneeze and she responded immediately with "shhh." She was very alert this whole day.

The last two days have been my play days. The winter weather was such that golf was not possible. Instead, the last two days were spent visiting some people from my old workplace of 21 years ago. It was enjoyable and time very well spent. The last visit was to the Veterans nursing facility where a senior work official has been staying for the past several months. He is bedridden, blind, and has no memory at all.

I spent some time talking with his spouse who is physically unable to care for him and lives in the mountains about 60 miles from the VA facility. She can only be with him a few days each week and then must return to their home. I have spent considerable time pondering their situation. I am so fortunate to be able to care for my Sweetheart here in our home and spend each day in her company.

During the last several days there are times when my Sweetheart just can't sit still in the wheel chair. She is constantly leaning forward, leaning back, or just trying to reposition herself in the chair. I have changed her diaper and every diaper change she is checked for sores and ointment is applied. Nothing has seemed to help. Today she just seemed very uncomfortable and kept shifting her weight. I put a small pillow behind her in the wheel chair and she seemed content. She never shifted her position again all afternoon. Sometimes it is the small and seemingly insignificant things that make a difference. Apparently she was trying to tell me something but I just wasn't listening.

It is the holiday season again. We have not decorated our home for the last several years and this year is no different. We have had lots of visitors coming to pay their respects. I have told people that the time to visit is between 4 and 6 PM any day because my Sweetheart will always be awake. She has seemed to respond well to the visitors. Mostly though, she ignores them but there are times when she does interact. Our daughter-in-law who lives in the local area was visiting and was ready to depart. She came to the work table and said goodbye. My Sweetheart responded with "don't take my clothes off." It was my guess that she thought our daughter-in-law was the hospice shower lady.

The regular caregiver who normally comes two days each week is taking time off during the holiday season. That means no play time for me but the weather is such that outside activities are not possible. I am definitely looking forward to my next time off and hopefully the weather will improve.

The holiday season has taken a toll. I put her on the scales today and she has gained 5 pounds in the last 10 days. I need to be more careful with her diet because weight gain is not good for either of us. I still plan to give her the sweet things that she enjoys so much but just limit the quantity. The extra weight definitely makes it more difficult for her to plant her good leg and stand.

Keeping her bowel movements regular seems to always be a challenge. Some time ago she was given one tablespoon of Miralax each morning. Then the amount of daily Miralax was reduced to one teaspoon daily and further reduced to one half teaspoon daily. Just recently her bowel movements have been extremely loose so the Miralax has been temporarily discontinued. She is still having at least one bowel movement daily. When she has two days without bowel movements she is given a suppository on the morning of the third day.

I often stop at thrift stores and look for something I can't live without. During a recent visit it was noted on one wall a small hand lettered sign indicating toys. Small plastic bags were displayed with small toys inside. I noticed one bag containing a hedgehog, a carrot, and a hotdog in a bun. They were stuffed toys that were made of a soft material. Each toy has a squeaker inside. My Sweetheart loves those toys but has never mastered the squeakers. I think they were a doggie toy but are a welcome addition to her table especially for the price.

When put into bed for the night or for naps, she never seems to move. She will be laying in exactly the same position as when she was placed in the bed. The bed has a side railing which is always raised to assure she doesn't fall. I have concluded that the reason she never moves is because she doesn't remember what she must do to move to her side or to her stomach.

We had visitors today. Our middle son and two of our smallest grandchildren arrived late in the evening after she was asleep for the night. The next morning when she saw our son, is was obvious that there was recognition. She greeted him with a big smile and a kiss. When the grandchildren came to say hello, they were greeted with a big kiss. She was happy and very alert during her waking hours. She didn't know the name of anyone but she knew they were family. She won't remember their visit after their return home but I'm convinced that she will have a recollection sometime in the future for just a moment.

Not much sleep last night for me. Finally at 3:40 AM I just gave up and got out of bed. I guess it is because of the anticipation of the events for today. Over 63 years ago was my high school graduation. Two classmates, husband and wife, live in the area and we are meeting to renew acquaintances. My Sweetheart is still sleeping soundly but my mind was just racing most of the night. Sleep just would not come. I'm sure it will be a memorable day and hopefully tonight will be a restful night.

My Sweetheart has had 11 bowel movements in the last 4 days. In the past she has been given miralax. The dosage has been reduced several times to only ½ teaspoon each day and then finally no miralax at all. The stools are not at all runny which eliminates diarrhea. This has been discussed with the nurse who could provide no insight as to the cause. I can only watch to see what comes next.

She doesn't know anyone and not even her own name but I'm convinced that at various times she has flashes of reality. It is so interesting to watch her and see the mannerisms surface periodically of the days gone by. They seem to only surface on rare occasions. She was sitting at her table working diligently and needed to cough. Her hand automatically covered her mouth while she was coughing. She is constantly looking in a mirror and adjusting some part of her hair. When being dressed with a pull-over blouse or sweater she needs no urging to pull the garment down around her waist.

She seldom smiles but today was a red letter day in that department. We had visitors and when she saw the first they were greeted with several very large smiles. A little later a daughter-in-law visited and again a big laugh and several very large smiles. She may go for days and never smile again.

During my last visit to my primary care doctor, she recommended that I obtain the book "Being Mortal" by Atul Gawande. He is a surgeon and it is one of several books that he has written. I have read it twice. It shows how the ultimate goal is not a good death but a good life—all the way to the very end. I would certainly recommend reading the book.

At 5:30 AM she was wide awake and it was apparent that she needed changing. After the new diaper she was again laid in the bed to rest. At 7 AM she was again wide awake. She was dressed, given her medications and breakfast. By 8:15 AM she was napping in her wheel chair. I'm hoping that her nap today will be a very long and restful nap. She just appeared to be very tired.

At 5 AM this morning she was wide awake and fussing. There was no BM but she was changed and moved to the kitchen for a drink, meds, and some breakfast. By 6:15 AM she was napping in her wheel chair so back to bed. Today is her shower day so by 9 AM she must be out of bed and ready to shower. This could end up being a 3 nap day. It will be interesting to see what else the day brings.

I was contacted by the Department of Administration to make a Meals on Wheels assessment. We have been receiving meals now for nearly one year and apparently they need to make sure we still qualify for the meals. After a lengthy question and answer period, I was informed that we still qualify to receive the meals.

She was awake early this morning and it was the beginning of the third day without a bowel movement. That means it is suppository day. I loosened the diaper and she immediately rolled to her right side and grabbed the bar at the foot of the master bed. That position on her right side is the position she takes when I'm cleaning her after a BM. Then I noticed that she'd had a small BM. I gave her a suppository and she finished her BM on the commode.

During her shower today I noticed a large brown mole on her right side just below her breast. It appeared to me that it was a melanoma cancer. When her nurse came a little later in the morning she examined it and agreed that it had all of the apparent characteristics of a melanoma. At this stage in her life, it doesn't seem appropriate to put her through any treatments of any kind. I decided to send her primary care doctor an email and ask her opinion on what should be done. I received a prompt response and she indicated that she would make a house call and examine the mole. She came after work and examined the mole and said that it was not a melanoma and was no problem. I couldn't believe that a doctor in this day would make a house call. She indicated that she was born in the wrong century that is why she made the house call. I told her that if I had a pig I would give it to her for the pay but instead just gave her a can of our special peaches.

Shingles again! Two days after noticing the suspected melanoma during her shower, it was noticed that she had a rash on her back. After close examination it appears to be another case of shingles. The hospice nurse came and confirmed my suspicions. My Sweetheart had a shingles shot but this is the third episode. The medication for treatment was delivered late in the evening with instructions to take one tablet 3 times daily for seven days. The tablets are 1000 mg and when ground and put into a liquid are extremely bitter. After trying the liquid approach, the preferred method is to grind up the tablet, sprinkled it on bread and smothered it with freezer jam.

My Sweetheart now has a terrible rash on her back. I think it is painful for her and is affecting her sleep patterns. The doctor advised that we should use cortisone ointment applied twice daily. I purchased the ointment and also the cortisone spray. It is surely easier to apply using the spray but the spray seems very upsetting during application. The ointment is applied after her shower on shower days. On non-shower days, her back is washed each morning and then the ointment is applied. After a full week of applying the ointment there seems to be some improvement in the rash and in her sleeping.

My Sweetheart's cousin from several hundred miles away came to visit. When she arrived, my Sweetheart was sleeping but awoke a short time later. During the process of changing her diaper and lifting her into the wheel chair, the cousin asked why I didn't have a Velcro back brace. For some reason the thought of securing a back brace had never entered my mind. I searched the internet and found a suitable back brace that arrived a few days later. Use of the back brace seems to have a definite benefit and makes the lifting seem easier.

It was 3 AM and my Sweetheart was awake and fussing. Her diaper was changed and she was back to sleep but not for long. At 4 AM she was wide awake and seemed to want to get out of bed. She was dressed, given her morning medications, and the breakfast meal. About 5:15 AM she was ready for a nap which lasted until 8 AM. The entire day was spent with long periods of being awake and only 1+ hour naps. Her total sleep time for the day was at least 4 hours less than normal. One of her medications is a low dose antibiotic to guard against urinary tract infections but I'm thinking maybe it isn't doing the job. Her temperature has been running close to 100 for several days now except when she was given Tylenol to reduce her fever. The hospice has been contacted and the supplies provided to take urine samples in an attempt to determine the problem.

Yes, it has been confirmed that she has a urinary tract infection. The hospice nurse called and said the medications would be delivered that afternoon. After a telephone call to the pharmacy, the delivery was finally made about 6 PM. The dosage is 3 capsules each day for seven days. The most difficult part of giving the medication is removing it from the capsules. In some cases, a toothpick must be used to remove the last of the medication. My Sweetheart readily takes the medication when sprinkled on bread with a liberal coating of jam.

She is still running a fever mostly in the PM. I suspected that the UTI medication was not effective. A new urine sample was taken and it tested negative for a UTI. Her sleep today was only 13 ½ hours at night and during the day she only napped for 1 ½ hours. Only 15 hours of sleep during a 24 hour period is the least amount of daily sleep in over 2 years.

My Sweetheart was sitting at her table and was fully engrossed in playing with her things. The television was on as usual and was showing a golfing commercial. She looked up just as the player hit the golf ball and she exclaimed "FORE". That is just another example of her having a moment of clarity.

I made a visit to the dollar store to get my Sweetheart some more colored beads. She now has 8 strands of beads with colors blue, red, white, and silver. The beads were intended for wearing around the neck but the strands were cut which makes them easier for her to handle. The beads are kept on her table in a small paper bowl. She is constantly playing with the beads along with other things. Apparently the bright colors attract her attention and make them her favorite.

There has been some improvement in the rash on her back but it isn't completely healed yet. I'm still using the cortisone ointment two times each day and have been for nearly a month now. The nurse will contact her doctor today to see if there may be another kind of ointment that will be more effective.

Since her UTI it seems that she has had some problems sleeping soundly at night. Several days ago, just before her bedtime, a small amount of night-time Nyquil was put in her drink. It seems to have a positive effect on her sleep. In my own case, a dose of the Nyquil before bedtime assures me that I will have a good and restful sleep.

Five weeks using the cortisone ointment and the rash is still there. The doctor asked if there had been any changes in the laundry soap used, shampoo, body wash or lotions. Since there were no changes she said to continue using the cortisone ointment two times each day. I certainly don't have much hope that things will improve very rapidly if at all.

We were given one large frozen brown trout. We always like fried trout and fried potatoes. That was one of our favorite meals. The trout had been filleted and most of the bones had been removed. I prepared it the same way that my Sweetheart always prepared it. Salt and pepper the trout and then roll it in flour. It was then fried in about half butter and half Crisco. We like it cooked to a golden brown. My Sweetheart really enjoyed both the trout and the fried potatoes. While she was eating, she suddenly stopped, reached to her mouth and carefully removed a small bone. She laid it on the side of the plate and then continued eating. It was clear that at that moment she knew just what she was doing and how to do it.

I woke her at 8 AM for her shower and had a terrible time getting her to take the morning medications. She ate almost nothing for breakfast and then would drink only ½ glass of juice. After the shower she went directly to bed for her nap that lasted over 6 hours. When she woke, she ate well and drank well but in just a short time after her meal she seemed exhausted. Visitors from our church came at 4 PM and she would only sit and doze in the wheel chair. I was able to get her to take the night medications without much problem but she was ready for bed at 5:30. Her total awake time today was only about 2 hours.

The terrible rash on her back just doesn't seem to get any better. We have been using the same ointment now for 6 weeks and her back just hasn't improved. She sleeps on the hospital bed with an air mattress. We use a protective pad over the sheets covering the area from her waist to her knees. The area above the protective pad has only a sheet covering the air mattress. I've had concerns that maybe too much heat is generated in that area which contributes to the rash. I have now covered that area with a cloth pad. She normally wears nylon underclothing on her upper body. Now the nylon underclothing has been removed and she wears only a cotton garment. Today I delivered a picture of the rash to her doctor and asked if there wasn't some ointment that would be more effective because the current medication just wasn't doing the job. Hopefully something can be prescribed that will be effective.

Last evening I was informed that the doctor had sent a new prescription to our pharmacy. We use three different pharmacies at various times. The prescription had been sent to the military mail order pharmacy rather than a local. The mail order pharmacy informed me that it would take 3-4 work days for processing, then preparation for mailing and then ultimately mailing. Normally the mail time is at least 3 days. Today is Friday, a week from Monday is a federal holiday so the medication would not be received for at least 10 days. At my request, the doctor sent a new prescription to a local pharmacy and it was delivered shortly after noon today.

I started using the new ointment in midafternoon on the day it arrived. I'm not sure what is happening but my Sweetheart was very restless at 5 AM and was wide awake at 6 AM. It was her third day with no bowel movement so it was suppository day. She had a good sized bowel movement in the commode then another an hour later and then still another an hour after that. She was put down for a nap after she was changed from the third bowel movement. I could see no apparent change in the appearance of the rash on her back. The doctor, in her email to me about the new prescription, indicated that the new ointment should be used once each day. The instructions on the prescription shows that it should be applied twice daily. It appears that I have a choice.

The Saturday before Memorial Day has been a time for gathering with my siblings. This began in 2002 after the death of my Mother. That day has always been set aside and I have made arrangements to attend. For some time now, I have had a feeling of uneasiness and that maybe I should not attend. It is now 5 days before the event and I still have not committed to attend. Caring for my Sweetheart is my number one priority. I would much rather forego attendance and be sorry for not attending than to attend and then be sorry for being away when I was needed most. This morning at 4:20 AM my Sweetheart was wide awake and needing care. As always, before that care can be given, I must put on my left knee brace. She was wide awake, her diaper was changed and she was fed an early breakfast. Before 6 AM she was tired and needed to be put down for a nap. Who knows, this may be a three nap day.

The rash on her back just doesn't seem to get any better. The hospice nurse took a picture of her back and showed it to the hospice doctor. He prescribed Prednisone tablets once a day for 5 days. We first started using over the counter Hydrocortisone cream. Then, the doctor prescribed Traimcinolone Acetonide cream which we are still using. Hopefully we can finally get some positive results.

Today the caregiver came and I had a day off. I was playing in another one of those seniors golf tourneys. I enjoy playing in them very much. The tourney was a one day affair and was located about 60 miles to the West. I needed to leave at 7 AM so I was up early and getting things around so I could leave. I went to the bedroom about 6:30 AM and my Sweetheart was wide awake. I know that she sensed that I was leaving. I changed her diaper, gave her the morning medications, gave her the morning drink and changed her narcotic pain patch before the caregiver arrived. As I looked back over the sleep records, she has seldom awoke that early in the morning. This is just another example that Alzheimer patients are more aware of their surroundings and events than they are given credit.

The nurse for my Sweethearts regular doctor called this afternoon and informed me that we now have another urinary tract infection and that a prescription had been sent to the local pharmacy that delivers. A little later in the day, I called the local pharmacy to make sure the delivery would be made today. They indicated that there was no record of any new prescription for my Sweetheart. A short time later the hospice nurse called with the same information and indicated that she had a copy of the prescription that had been sent to the pharmacy. She faxed the copy to the pharmacy and the medication was delivered at 7 PM.

And thus has ended the ninth day.

CHAPTER 10

The Tenth Day

It was Wednesday and one of my weekly days off. It started like most Wednesdays where my Sweetheart is awakened about 8 AM in preparation for her shower. I left at about nine and went straight to the golf course for a leisurely game of golf. The weather was great, the golf course was great and the pace of play was great. After the round of golf and some lunch it was still only 2:30 PM with my curfew being at 4 PM. There were no errands to run so I just went straight home. My Sweetheart was still sleeping from the nap that had started a little after 9 AM. She continued to sleep until nearly 4 PM. She had eaten the breakfast meal at 8 AM so it had been a full 8 hours since her last meal. I am extremely concerned that we are now entering the last days.

It seems that some days she is extremely alert and then there are days when she is far away in another place. She usually sits at her table and is constantly moving and handling her things. The beads seem to be her favorite now with the way they feel and the many difference colors. Lately though she just doesn't seem to even notice them. It was 3:20 AM she had a large bowel movement and needed changing. It was accomplished quite rapidly but she had a difficult time going back to sleep. She woke at 8:15 this morning and it was difficult getting her to take her medications. Within an hour she was dozing in her wheel chair. Her weight at the last weight check was three pounds less than the previous week. I'm not sure what to expect during these next few days.

The hospice doctor prescribed a different medication for the rash on her back. The new ointment is to be applied twice daily for 14 days. The hospice nurse delivered the medication in the afternoon so the first application was made just before her bedtime. She just wasn't alert at all today. There was difficulty in getting her to eat and take her medications. She awoke this morning at 8:15 AM and after her medications and breakfast she was ready for a nap at 9:15 AM. That nap lasted for 6 ¼ hours making her total sleep time for the day just over 21 hours. Not a good day that is for sure.

At times it is an effort to keep things straight between the hospice doctor and her regular doctor. I never have talked with the hospice doctor but the hospice nurse talks with him regularly. When I have an issue that is not related to her hospice her regular doctor is contacted. There are times when both doctors may respond a few days apart but are responding to the same issue. I try to keep her regular doctor informed by email.

I decided that it was time to take my Sweetheart on an automobile ride. I made the necessary preparations and moved her to the garage. Her wheel chair was placed as close to the seat as was possible and I lifted and turned her to try and sit her on the edge of the seat. For some reason she just wasn't helping that much with the standing and she slid off the seat down to the lower door shelf. Again I lifted her to the edge of the seat but she just couldn't help at all and slid to the lower door shelf again. I decided to abandon the idea and put her back into the wheel chair. When I lifted her, she didn't plant her good leg as usual and with great difficulty she was seated on the very edge of the wheel chair. It seems she is getting more and more difficult for me to lift and automobile rides are just a thing in the past.

She just didn't want to wake up this morning. I tried several different approaches but none seemed to work. It is her shower day and the normal wake up time is 8:15 AM. When I changed her, the diaper was hardly wet after 14 ½ hours of sleep. She wouldn't drink any juice. Finally, I took a small teaspoon of freezer jam and was able to put it into her mouth. It was very hard to give the morning medications but it was finally accomplished. She did eat a small amount but not without considerable effort on my part. The rash on her back seems to be worse today than it has been for several days. I contacted a dermatologist and inquired about an appointment or possibly a house call. I was told that the doctor or a representative would contact me.

No response from the doctor concerning the calls that were made yesterday. Late this afternoon a delivery was made by a local pharmacy of yet another ointment for her back. I did not recognize the name of the prescribing doctor but the ointment is for her back and is to be applied twice daily for 14 days. The fourteen day cycle for the last ointment was completed this morning. Hopefully we will get some positive results from this medication.

She seems to be eating and drinking a little better now. Her back has shown some improvement but is not completely healed. Some days she is quite responsive but other days she just sits and stares. I talk to her constantly while I'm caring for her. Mostly there is no response but at times she will make a one word response that is not really appropriate. For example, I may ask her if she would like a drink and she will respond "no" but then takes the straw and drinks most of the glassful. She does continue to have a good disposition and it is very satisfying for me to be able to give her care.

Lately I've been pondering what I will do with myself when she is gone. It is hard to imagine how empty my life will be without her to care for. When people ask me what I'll do with my time, my response is that maybe I'll just go walking down at the indoor mall. In reality I can't think of a thing that would be more distasteful than walking at the mall. I continue to do my own lawn and to care for the wooded area at the back of our property. I'm often asked why I don't hire someone to do that work but I do need something to do with my time. Really there is no use dwelling on what I will do because it will be somewhat like things are now, no plan but just take things one day at a time and one hour at a time.

I recently received an unsolicited magazine. As I thumbed through the pages there were several notes at the bottom of pages that read "Walk to End Alzheimer's." A few pages later in the magazine there was a full page with a heading "The end of Alzheimer's starts with you."

One of the captions at the bottom of the page reads "The disease is all around us, but the power to stop it is within us." In my opinion, those captions and comments are nonsense. A bunch of people walking down the road will do nothing to end Alzheimer's.

My Sweetheart was wide awake at 6:30 this morning with a large bowel movement. I was very relieved because for the last two weeks her only bowel movements were induced by suppositories. She was alert and ready to begin another day but after a little more than an hour she was ready to start a six hour nap. Her sleep time is gradually increasing each month and for the last three months the average sleep time has been over 19 hours each day. Most of the time she eats well and her weight has remained quite stable between 127 and 130 pounds.

I woke her this morning at 8:15 in preparation for her shower. She was very tired and was sleeping in her wheel chair at 9:15. A short time later she was napping and was still napping at 4 PM when I woke her again. She was not alert at all and while sitting at her table she didn't even touch the beads and other items on the table. The total sleep time for the day was 20 ¾ hours. There is not much time left for eating and other activities. I'm fearful that the end of my care giving may be getting much closer. I'm surely not prepared for the end.

Her back is now completely healed. It has been a long process of trial and error. We completed the 14 day cycle and a small amount of the ointment remained which was used beyond the 14 days. The nurse suggested that medicated talcum powder be applied to her back after her shower and before bedtime. Hopefully it will be of benefit to prevent further rashes.

Yesterday morning she had a very large bowel movement. Last night at about 10:30 PM she had another large bowel movement. Then again this morning at 6:30 AM yet another. That many bowel movements are quite uncharacteristic for her. I'm wondering if this is going to be the routine for the coming days.

The Nurse Practitioner from the hospice called and needed an appointment. The time has come for recertification of my Sweetheart for the hospice program. She had a lot of questions and took her vital signs. At the conclusion of her visit my question was does she still qualify. Her response was definitely, she will not get any better. From the records that I keep it is easy to see that she has definitely declined in the last two months.

My Sweetheart was still sleeping at 11 this morning so I woke her for breakfast. By noon, she had eaten and was dozing in her wheelchair. She was laid in the hospital bed for a nap and was still sleeping at 4 PM. I woke her and fed her the dinner meal. Her total sleep time for today was 21 ¼ hours. Last month she averaged 19.4 hours of sleep each day. There surely isn't much awake time to give her medications twice daily and to feed her the meals.

This morning she awoke at about 9 and was very alert. Shortly after her breakfast meal she was dozing in her wheel chair so it was back into her bed for a nap. When she awoke some 4 hours later she was again very alert. As she was eating her meal she looked at me and exclaimed "I love you." I was somewhat shocked and amused. Yes, today was a very good day.

My Sweetheart seems to enjoy visitors. We don't have a lot of visitors but we do have people coming several times each week. The shower lady, the hospice CNA, comes three times each week and the hospice nurse comes twice weekly. Additionally, the hospice spiritual person every two weeks and the hospice social worker comes once each month. The missionaries from our church are regular weekly visitors. I try to position my Sweetheart directly in front of the visitors so she has direct eye contact with them. At times there will be some interaction with them but other times she will just sit and stare. I do know that at times she does get some enjoyment from the visits.

A recent article in the Time magazine entitled "Untangling Alzheimer's" was read with interest. It is apparent to me that not much progress is being made on prevention and treatment. This particular article suggests that lifestyle changes may help protect the brain as you age. It also suggests that natural interventions appear to have powerful effects on areas of the brain that are vulnerable to aging. I'm sure the words were carefully chosen because the bottom line is—they don't really know but it makes good reading.

My Sweetheart has a shower three days each week, Monday, Wednesday and Friday. The established time for the shower for nearly 18 months has been about 9:15 AM. Last Friday our regular shower lady was called to provide shower assistance in another area and didn't arrive until 12:30 PM. The next Monday, without any notice, she didn't arrive until 3 PM. Today, Wednesday, I received a telephone call at 8:30 AM that a different shower lady would be coming and she would arrive at 10:30 AM. It was my day off so I relayed the information to the lady who cares for my Sweetheart on my off days. When I returned I was informed that the substitute shower lady would be coming again on Friday and would arrive about 1 PM or if I didn't like that she could come at 5:15 AM. When I called the office to tell them neither time was acceptable, they informed me that our regular shower lady had terminated her employment and the substitute would become the regular shower lady.

Friday morning came and I had not received any information concerning what to expect for timing of the shower. The nurse arrived for her Friday visit at the normal time and informed me that we would have a different shower lady and that she would arrive at about the normal times. After we discussed the events surrounding the change, it was apparent that the nurse had interceded on our behalf to assure that we had our desired shower time.

Our current shower lady has been doing this kind of work for 23 years. She told of a lady patient who for some reason is afraid of showers which makes her work very difficult. This past week it became extremely difficult and she asked her husband if he had some gum. He gave her a stick of gum and she gave it to the patient to chew. Immediately the patient became very calm and the shower was completed without any further difficulty. She explained to her husband that we have used gum for a very long period of time with the same result. It may not work for everyone but it is worth trying because it does work for some people.

Yesterday my Sweetheart was very tired. Her normal bedtime is 6 PM but last night she was put into bed at 5 PM. She was still sleeping at noon so a short time later I woke her. She ate a good meal and then was extremely sleepy again. She was put into bed for a nap and again

I had to wake her just after 4 PM. Her total sleep time for today was 22 ¼ hours.

She normally eats and drinks very well especially in the mornings. Today that was not the case. She would only drink a small amount and it was very difficult to get her to eat the bread and jam with the crushed morning medications. Finally, I primed her with a few candy skittles and then was able to finish the medications and she ate a small breakfast. It worries me that we may be entering a new era of not eating well.

The last few days it seems that she is very congested when she awakes in the morning. She will cough with a very noticeable croupy sound. It just doesn't sound good to me. The nurse frequently checks her lungs but nothing is noted. I have now started raising the head of the bed considerably when she is sleeping during the night and for naps.

Each year our middle son insists that he wants to play a two man best ball golf tourney with his dad. I tell people that he thinks it may be his last chance before I croak. Well, this past weekend was the time for the annual tourney. He travelled some 400 miles with part of his family and arrived late on Friday night. Two of his daughters in their early 20's are CNA's and working on nursing degrees. They were charged with caring for my sweetheart. Since we had to leave home for the tourney early, my regular paid caregiver consented to come for 3 hours the first morning and give them instruction on how we do things. The second day my Sweetheart did not sleep all that much but was very alert and talking. I know at times she did recognize some of our visitors. I think her lack of sleep was because of the excitement she felt with all the visitors and the extra attention that she received. When the family left to return home and things became quiet she was immediately ready for bed. It was a good weekend – and we won the tourney.

Yesterday I woke my Sweetheart at 8 AM, gave her the morning medications, and fed her breakfast. It was her shower day and immediately following the shower, she was laid in the hospital bed for her morning nap. The caregiver came and I departed to participate in a golf tourney with a late start. I returned home about 7 in the evening and of course she was asleep for the night. Today I left at 7:15 AM to participate in day two of the golf tourney. I returned home just after 3 PM. She was still sleeping from her afternoon nap. As I sat waiting for her to awaken, it struck me that I hadn't seen my Sweetheart awake or been able to talk with her for over 30 hours. I had a feeling of emptiness and continued to check on her every few minutes until she was awake. I have no idea if she missed me but I surely missed her.

When she is lifted to a standing position she plants her left leg and bears most of her own weight. Although she only weighs 126, an old guy like me could never lift her total weight. Of late I have noted it seems more difficult to lift her and at times she bears hardly any weight on her left leg. When that occurs she is reseated and lifted again in hopes that she will bear more weight on her left leg making my job easier to accomplish. I'm sure that as things progress my task will not become any easier. I just take things one day at a time and sometimes one hour at a time.

I awoke this morning at 2:47 AM to a terrible smell. It was one of those very messy bowel movements. She was cleaned, put on a new pull-up diaper and she was laid down in the hospital bed so she could continue her sleep. I'm always careful to put on my left knee brace before I start lifting. This morning at 8 AM another huge bowel movement. I have been giving her a very small dose of Miralax one time each day but definitely not today. She was given two anti-diarrhea tablets with her morning medications. Her normal dosage of Miralax has been two teaspoons each day. I plan to skip at least one and maybe two days but when the dosage is resumed, it will be only one teaspoon each day.

Today is Monday and it is her shower day so I awoke her early. The nurse came at the regular time on Monday and informed me that she has too many patients and was wondering if I objected to a different nurse being assigned. My response was no I don't mind but no male nurse. I just do not want a male nurse caring for my Sweetheart. A few minutes later a telephone call informing me that the regular shower lady was not available this morning and a substitute would be coming at the normal time. This hospice is very good at keeping me informed when there are changes and the changes don't come very often.

Our yearly supply of peaches was delivered today. We became aware of a small cannery in Oregon that cans peaches and they taste just like those my Mother canned. Their peaches are not available in any grocery store in this area but once each year they deliver orders. After the delivery was complete, one of the truck drivers indicated that this was just a part time job for him because his regular job was working in a memory care unit. I immediately began asking questions about how things were done where he works. I showed him the rotating and sliding shower bench. He couldn't believe such an item was available and expressed several times how great it would be for the patient as well as the caregiver. I also showed him my Sweethearts activity table. Again, he had never seen one in use and marveled on how effective he thought it would be.

Our shower lady was talking about some of her in-home care patients. She indicated that I wouldn't believe some of the things that she sees in some homes. In many instances the people providing the care have no interest in caring for the patients and are forced into being caregivers. Apparently the inability to afford moving them to a care facility is the driving factor. In our case, moving my Sweetheart to a care facility was never considered. I am fortunate to have a Sweetheart with a good disposition and also have the ability to provide the necessary care. I would never be critical of another person unless I had walked in their moccasins and faced all of the problems and issues that they have faced.

I woke her at the normal time for a shower day but she just couldn't seem to get fully awake. I moved her into the kitchen to give her the morning drink and her medications but she just was not responsive at all. She wouldn't eat and wouldn't drink. The hospice nurse was here at the time and she had no suggestions but asked if this was a normal occurrence. Finally, I just gave up and sat at her side trying to hold her head erect as she slept in the wheel chair. A short time later she started to arouse and opened her eyes. I was successful in getting her to drink the majority of her juice and to eat her bread and jam with the crushed morning medications. It took significant effort to get her to eat a small bowl of fruit. The shower lady arrived just as she was finishing the fruit.

We did give her a shower and then put her into bed. Hopefully, she will awake rested and able to eat a normal meal.

It was just a normal shower day and she was awakened at about 8 AM. The nurse arrived a short time later and completed her visit. My helper arrived at 9 AM and I was off to a local golf course. When I returned a short time after 3 PM, my helper informed me that she waited and waited for the shower lady to come. Finally, about 9:30 AM she took my Sweetheart to the bathroom to start her shower. She finished the shower and put her in the hospital bed for a nap because she was completely exhausted. Finally, about 11:30 AM, someone from the hospice call and said the regular shower lady had not come to work that day but someone would come to give a shower about 1:30 PM. They were informed that there was no need because the shower had already been given. The normal shower time for my Sweetheart is between 8:45 and 9:15 AM. It is understandable that at times and for various reasons employees will not come to work. When that happens, a simple telephone call before the scheduled time of the visit should be made. The local hospice office was visited and I expressed my dissatisfaction with how things were handled in our case.

Today was a sleepy day for my Sweetheart. She didn't wake this morning until just before noon. After she had eaten her breakfast meal it was nap time which lasted until 4 PM. Her total sleep time for today was 22 ½ hours which is a new record. She is apparently making up for yesterday when she slept just over 18 hours.

When the nurse came the last time she was given a urine sample from my Sweetheart. After it was analyzed the results were sent to her regular doctor. It was determined that she needed to be treated with antibiotics. I was asked where the prescription should be sent and I gave them the name of the local pharmacy used by our hospice. As I was reviewing my credit card purchases on the computer and noted that there was a charge by the pharmacy for the antibiotics. I questioned the nurse because always in the past those kinds of medications have been covered by the hospice. It was an error by the pharmacy and they are in the process of reversing the charge.

It was another sleepy day for my Sweetheart. I woke her just before noon and gave her the morning medications and her breakfast. She was very tired in a short time and napped again until 4 PM. Today was a 22 ½ hour sleep day for her. Two days in a row of sleeping over 22 hours worries me that we may be coming to her last days. The nurses have warned me that she will just sleep more and more. There is hardly time to give her medications and feed her a meal before she is asleep in her chair. I know we are on borrowed time. Today marked her 44th month as a hospice patient.

The local newspaper today had a large article talking about care giving. At the beginning of the article it indicated that November is National Family Caregiver Month. Here I have been a caregiver for a long time and I didn't even know that. The article talked about many things and one of intense interest to me was caring for oneself. At one point it indicated that caregivers should do "Mindfulness Meditation which is a form of relaxation which helps reconnect a person with their body by sitting in any comfortable space and redirecting the mind from the stress of the day to an awareness of each part of the body by stages." I read and reread that passage and just got more confused. I thought of the many military schools that I have attended in the past and it always seemed the particular subject had a "school solution". The instructors would tell us to remember the school solution for the test but then forget it because it doesn't work in the real world. They would then go on and expound on the real world and practical solution. In my opinion mindfulness meditation is a school solution which has absolutely no practical application to caregivers in the real world.

The last few days have been very interesting. It seems that keeping her bowel movements regular is a constant effort. When she doesn't have a BM for two days in a row it is suppository time. I haven't used a suppository for some time now. Two days ago it was a 2 BM day. The next day it was a 3 BM day and the Miralax was stopped that morning. Today, another no Miralax day, she woke with a huge BM. Hopefully she will become somewhat stable on her BM's.

A lady from our church called and wanted to come and visit my Sweetheart. In the past she had a church assignment to visit her regularly but that changed and she hasn't been here in some time. When she arrived she brought a small plastic container filled with peeled apple slices. My Sweetheart seemed to really enjoy them. After they were all eaten, I peeled and sliced several apples and put them in a container. The next morning they were starting to turn brown. I'm not very smart on what to do to prevent that but my son said they needed a slight coating of lemon juice. Not having any lemon juice available, they were coated with orange juice and it worked, the brown on the slices disappeared.

Our family always gathers for Thanksgiving. This year was no different except when one son arrived with eight of his family and three visitors, we had a houseful. My Sweetheart seemed to respond quite well to the all of our visitors. On Thanksgiving morning she was awaken a little early and then laid down for a nap. Our dinner was set for 1 PM so she was awakened at 12:30 but just would not open her eyes. She was moved into the room with 16 other people but still would not open her eyes. Before the meal we took a group picture and then pictures of several smaller groups. She was moved to the table but was still sleeping in her wheel chair. Finally after several attempts, I was able to get a small amount of her favorite salad into her mouth. The instant she tasted the salad her eyes came open and she was eager to eat the remainder of her meal.

Twenty seven years ago we remodeled our kitchen and installed all new appliances. We have a built-in double door refrigerator/freezer with wood panel doors that match our cabinetry. Two days after Thanksgiving it stopped working. The repair people were called the next regular workday and they responded with a same day visit. The unit was purchased and installed in November 1990. My greatest fear was that it could not be repaired and would need to be replaced. Of course, nothing is available that would accommodate our wood paneling. The technician quickly diagnosed the problem and determined that the necessary parts should be available. His estimate for repair was in approximately five days. We have at least another five days of living out of coolers but that is the least of our worries.

Today was my day off and also her shower day. I woke her just before 9, gave her the morning drink and her medications. My helper arrived at

9 and fed her the breakfast meal. The shower lady was just a little later than expected so my Sweetheart was laid in the bed until she arrived. After the shower she was very tired so it was back to bed for a nap. I arrived home a little early and she was still sleeping. Finally at 5 PM she was awakened but was never fully awake. She was fed the lunch meal with great difficulty, given the night medications with great difficulty and put into bed for the night. She seemed completely exhausted and was in a deep sleep as soon as she laid her head on the pillow. Being the last day of the month her average sleep time each day was computed and the result was 20.0 hours per day sleeping. That is an increase of ½ hour per day from last month. However, she did gain 2 pounds this past month but of course this was a holiday month.

Would you believe it, another urinary tract infection (UTI). There was no specific sign but she just didn't seem to be doing that well. I monitor her temperature each time she awakens and it seemed to be elevated to some degree. This morning I had the feeling that a urine sample should be taken and tested before the weekend arrived. The medication was delivered by the nurse later in the day and the first tablet was given with the regular night medication. Two tablets per day for seven days are the instructions.

She took the medications over the weekend and late Monday afternoon the nurse called and said to stop the medication she had been taking. Apparently this UTI needs a different medication. The prescription has been sent to the pharmacy but no medications delivered yet to today. Not good! Four days have been wasted in treating her UTI with the wrong medication.

I woke her at 11 AM today and started the new medication. She seemed very tired and it was difficult getting her to take the morning medications. She ate very little breakfast and was put back into bed. I woke her at 3 PM to give her some lunch and the mid-day UTI medication. Again, it was very difficult getting her to take the medication and she ate very little of the lunch. She was extremely tired so it was back into bed for more napping. She was awakened at 5 PM and her night medications were crushed and put in a small dish with two tablespoons of soft strawberry jam. The medications and jam were thoroughly mixed. She ate the mixture without hesitation. She ate a very small amount and it was back to bed at 6 PM for the night. This has been a difficult day and I'm very concerned.

We are in the middle of a cold spell. We are having sub-zero temperatures at night and low teens during the day. My greatest fear has happened. I've gotten a terrible cold. I have some face masks which I wear when she is awake because I have to be around her. I'm trying all kinds of cold medicine but nothing seems to help. Someone told me if you go to a doctor for a cold, it will take seven days to get well. If you don't go to a doctor, you will get well in a week.

I had a regular visit to the dermatologist today and took a picture of my Sweetheart's back when she had the terrible rash. When the doctor entered the room the picture of her back was laying on my jacket. He immediately asked if that was my back. I explained that it was a picture of my wife's back and I had tried to get an appointment for her but couldn't because she wasn't a patient. His response was that shouldn't make any difference, she's family. He indicated that in the future if she needed an appointment I may need to call his personal cell phone number.

My Sweetheart had been put into bed for the night and about an hour later it was apparent she needed her diaper changed. It was a huge BM and really quite messy to get her changed. During the entire time, she just didn't awaken. When it was time to put on a clean diaper she wouldn't stand or assist in any way. Finally, a tape-on diaper was used and put on her as well as it could be under the circumstances. When everything was completed she was covered and still laid peacefully sleeping. She was checked various times during the night and was still laying in the same position the following morning.

The normal wake up time on shower mornings is 8 AM. Today she just wouldn't wake up. I managed to get her to drink a full glass of juice but could not get her to take her medicine on bread and jam. She wouldn't take even one bite of her breakfast so I just gave up and laid her back in the bed to sleep. When the shower lady came she was awakened, given the shower and dressed. She was taken to the kitchen and given the morning medications and her breakfast. After the last bite she was sound asleep in her wheel chair. The hospice nurse indicated that she believes that the "transition" has begun. I guess that is the term they use to indicate that she is getting ready to die. I have certainly made lots of preparation for that day but I'm not nearly ready for it to come. We shall see what the remainder of today and the rest of the week bring.

I don't believe my Sweetheart is ready to transition yet. Yes, she does sleep a lot with the average for last month being 20.6 hours each day. That is an increase of over half an hour from last month. Her weight stayed very stable though and most of the time she eats and drinks with no problems. With that amount of sleep each day there isn't much time remaining for other activities. She seldom stays awake for much over an hour at a time.

I believe it is time to get a urine sample and check for a urinary tract infection. The last two times I've gotten urine samples they have been contaminated so the lab didn't test them further. I stopped by the hospice office today and told them we need to get a clean sample and apparently the nurse will have to do that. She is supposed to visit tomorrow with the necessary supplies to insert a catheter to get the sample. My Sweetheart's behavior seems just a little strange and I'm grasping for reasons. I hope that getting the sample will not be too uncomfortable for her.

Well, getting a clean urine sample failed miserably. The nurse tried and tried but was unable to get a catheter inserted. I'm convinced that the only way that can happen is to put my Sweetheart under sedation. I'm also convinced that putting her under sedation to obtain a urine sample will not happen especially with her being a hospice patient. I do have four days of a UTI medication on hand and started giving it immediately following the failed catheter attempt. She seemed quite upset the remainder of the day. During her second nap, she had a huge bowel movement that was the messiest of all time. She was covered from her knees to her navel on both the front and back side. The following day was a disaster day. She didn't sleep well, she didn't eat well and she just seemed very upset all day. She woke up that morning at 7 AM which is the earliest wakeup in over a year. Her average sleep time for that day was almost 3 hours less than normal. The attempted catheter was just a very traumatic experience for her and we won't do that again.

I was at the grocery store and remembered that there were times when my Sweetheart really enjoyed thousand island salad dressing. On an impulse, I bought a bottle. One of the meals on wheels was some kind of chicken and potato mixture and it wasn't really all that appetizing. I mixed some thousand island dressing and she ate every bite. Today her meal was roast beef with mashed potatoes and gravy. Again, I used some thousand island dressing on the roast beef and she seemed to really enjoy it. I need to keep a supply of the dressing available.

Today was my Sweetheart's 78th birthday and It was a busy day. The hospice folks brought her some birthday flowers, a card and some goodies. Then, she was visited by four different groups. None called in advance but just came and my Sweetheart was wide awake during every visit. I know that she enjoyed the day and all the attention.

It seems that the hospice nurse and the shower lady believe my Sweetheart is showing some agitation and anxiety during her showers. They believe that she needs some kind of calming medication. I really don't see a need but have consented to a trial. The doctor prescribed Alprazolam in a very low dose. Next shower day I'll give her a tablet along with her regular medications. By chance, I had an appointment with the prescribing doctor and we discussed the need. She gave me some specific instructions and indicated that if there were any undesirable effects at all to discontinue immediately.

It is shower day and the first day for the new medication. Her breakfast was prepared, her drink was warmed and her morning medications, including the new medication, was mixed with applesauce. I went to awaken her and she just didn't want to wake-up. She was sat-up on the edge of the bed and when I attempted to lift her and pull up her clean diaper, her good leg just collapsed. I managed to get her back onto the edge of the bed and the second lift the leg collapsed again but I managed to get her to the edge of the wheel chair. The next attempt to pull up the diaper failed and she ended up sitting on the floor. She wouldn't drink, she wouldn't eat but I was successful in getting her to take the morning medications. She was showered and put back into bed.

And thus ended the tenth day.

CHAPTER 11

The Eleventh Day

The hospice nurse has been warning me that she believes that my Sweetheart is beginning to transition. I've chosen to ignore those warnings but today they just can't be ignored any longer. Her breakfast this morning consisted of one-fourth glass of orange juice, maybe one bite of pancake, and about one-fourth cup of applesauce with her crushed medications. After sleeping over 14 hours, she was laid in her bed about 9 AM and slept until 8 AM the following day. Her last full meal was over 37 hours ago. She has had those long sleeping spells in the past but they would always be preceded by a good breakfast. I talked with the nurse before she departed and she asked if I had read the pamphlet "When Death is Near", a caregiver's guide. Over two years ago when I changed to this hospice, they had furnished a binder full of information. At that time I did read all of the information but after the nurse left today I refreshed my memory. I was constantly checking to see if she is awake and asking if she would like to have something to eat or drink. Of course, there is was no response. I talked with our three sons and informed them of the latest developments. One of our sons came to our home and spent part of the evening with us. His visit certainly made the evening easier for me.

It was difficult for me to sleep last night and I was constantly checking to see if she was still breathing. About 8 this morning she started to stir and it wasn't long until she was wide awake. Naturally she was thirsty and hungry and ate a very good breakfast. The day was a little unusual because it was a three nap day for her. I'm thinking that the reason for nearly 24 hours of uninterrupted sleep was because of the new medication, Alprazolam. I don't intend to use that medication again but if I should it would be only a partial dose. The shower lady is not very happy with me. She believes that my Sweetheart's behavior during shower makes her work more difficult. I've never agreed with that except she does try at times to stand. I plan to use a gait belt as a seat belt to prevent her from standing.

It was shower day again today and of course, none of the new medication was given. She woke a little early and ate a good breakfast. Within an hour she was dozing in her wheel chair and was put back into bed. She napped until shower time, was awakened, showered and put back into bed. She had a good long nap and when she awoke was very alert. She ate a large evening meal and was awake and alert for almost two hours.

After the 37 hour sleep, I became concerned about final arrangements should she pass away. The obituary has been updated. The funeral program has been reviewed. I arbitrarily chose two songs for the funeral and the lady who will help me with the music has indicated that she wasn't familiar with either. My Sweetheart planned two funerals, her parents. Her father passed away first and one of the songs that I had picked was sang at his funeral. The other song that I picked was sang at her mother's funeral. Now I know that I have selected the right songs for my Sweetheart's funeral.

The weather for some time now has been terrible and all of the golf courses are covered with over a foot of snow. During my free days I have visited several memory care facilities just to find out how they operated, the staffing and the cost. Most of the facilities cost in the neighborhood of $5,000 per month. The last facility that was visited charges $6,200 per month for the level of care needed for my Sweetheart. I have never seriously considered putting her in a care facility. However, should it become necessary that I have knee replacement surgery it could become necessary for a short period of time.

She has just completed her 47th month as a hospice patient. At the close of this last month her average sleep time each day was 20.9 hours which is an increase over the preceding month. She is also weighed at the end of each month and her weight was 123 pounds, a loss of 3 pounds this month. I see some definite changes and only hope that when the time comes that she goes easily rather than prolonged suffering.

It seems that her awake time is getting shorter and shorter. Seldom can she stay awake for a full hour between naps. Twenty one or more hours of sleep each day has become the norm. Frequently she is given her night medications immediately following her last meal of the day. Most days she is laid down for the night close to 5 PM. Spending so much time in bed can cause bed sores but so far we have been very fortunate and haven't had to cope with that problem.

Last evening she was just very anxious and didn't seem to want to settle down after being put into bed for the night. She was constantly pushing the covers down and then feeling cold. This seemed to go on all during the night and I must have covered her at least half a dozen times. My first thought was that maybe she has another urinary tract infection and was considering getting a urine sample. This afternoon though she was sleeping very soundly and appeared to be doing the same as she did during the night.

Shower day is on Monday, Wednesday and Friday. The hospice nurse comes on Monday and Friday just before the shower lady. On Wednesday the shower lady has a morning meeting and we are never sure of her arrival time. This past Wednesday, a day off for me, I told my helper to just leave my Sweetheart sleeping until the shower lady arrives. After the shower she could then be given her morning medications and the meal. She indicated that it worked very well. It was my intention to do the same on Friday and just leave her sleeping. The nurse can take the vital signs while she is sleeping and then we would wake her for the shower. Just before 8 AM, I noticed that she had a bowel movement and needed changing and of course during the changing she became fully awake. The nurse had significant difficulty taking the vital signs because the automatic blood pressure machine would not display a reading. Finally, she resorted to the old fashioned way and got a reading of 84/40. She also indicated that her heart beat was very faint. She ate well and after the shower was put into bed for her nap which lasted from

9 AM until 4:15 PM. I had difficulty getting her fully awake so she could be fed another meal and given the night medications. Her total sleep time for the day was 22 ¼ hours.

This morning she was awakened at 10:15 and given her morning medications and a good meal. Within 45 minutes she was dozing in her wheel chair and ready for her nap. The hospice spiritual person was coming at 4 PM today so I woke her at 3:45 and planned to feed her the evening meal and give the night medications. She just didn't want to wake up. I tried various things to no avail. I was able to get her to drink nearly ½ glass of juice but no night medications or food. Finally, I just gave up and put her back into bed. It sounded like she may have some congestion in her lungs or maybe it was just something in her throat. Yesterday, I had discussed with the hospice nurse my desire to have someone make me a video of me caring for her as well as some of the hospice people doing their work. I definitely think that would be something that I would treasure but maybe I've waited too long.

I checked my Sweetheart at 6:30 PM and she was partially awake. I raised the head of the bed and gave her some applesauce with her night medications. She seemed hungry and ate it very well. Her diaper was changed and she was fed a light evening meal and seemed quite alert. It wasn't long though until she was ready to go to sleep for the night. I guess that the earlier experience was because she just wasn't ready to end her nap.

Today was my Sweetheart's anniversary. Four years ago today she was placed in the hospice program. At that time I certainly didn't think she would be with us 4 years later. Some days I think the end may be near but other days she seems to be doing well. She has a grip like iron and I have bruises on both arms and hands caused by her grip. Of course, I do bruise easily. At the end of this last month she had averaged 21.1 hours of sleep each day and her weight was 123 pounds. The weight keeps going down slightly each month and the average sleep time increases.

The last several weeks it seems that she is just more and more difficult to get fully awake and that results in difficulty getting her to eat. I have informed the hospice nurse that I believe she is declining rapidly. Today was completely different though, she was so wide awake and alert, it was almost unbelievable. She ate extremely well and seemed to respond with one word answers to most questions. It certainly is an interesting journey and I have a lot of special memories.

I received a telephone call from the Meals on Wheels people. I was informed that it was annual recertification time and the rules had changed in some areas. My Sweetheart no longer qualifies for meals seven days each week. On the days when I have caregiver help so I can leave the house, those days are non-qualifying days. That means that on Wednesdays and Thursdays of each week she is not entitled to meals. We definitely rely on those meals and when I was informed that we would get meals for only five days each week, they were told that I would like to start receiving the meals on wheels for myself assuming that I qualified. I also qualify for meals on five days of each week so the bottom line is that instead of us receiving only seven meals each week, we will now be receiving ten meals. The meals freeze well and are easy to thaw and prepare.

This morning was shower day and I planned to wake her, give her the morning medications and breakfast before the shower. She just didn't want to wake up. She did take the morning medications in applesauce, drank a small amount of juice but not even one bite of food. After her shower, she was so tired that food was not an option. She was put into bed for a nap and at 2 PM, five hours later, I attempted to wake her again. She was just too tired but did drink a very small amount of juice and one bite of food. She was put back into bed and at 4:15 PM she was awake, hungry and thirsty. I worried all afternoon but in the end there was no need to worry. She just wasn't ready to wake up and eat.

Another month has ended and her average sleep time for this month ended up at 21.4 hours. That sure doesn't leave much time for eating and other activities. This was her shower day and I left her sleeping until they were ready to put her into the shower. She was awakened at 8:30 AM, showered, then I gave her the morning medications plus some food and juice. She just wasn't interested in eating or drinking but I finally did get her to take some food. She ended up back in bed at 9:15 AM. She hardly moved all day and at 5 this afternoon she was still sleeping. I managed to get her awake and into the kitchen but she was just too tired to eat or drink much of anything. Finally in desperation, I gave her some frosted animal cookies and she did eat those. I guess that primed the pump because after the cookies she ate a good meal and drank a normal amount of juice. It seems that it is getting more and more difficult to get her to eat a decent meal. These are definitely not good signs but they are to be expected.

5 AM and she is fussing in her bed. She had a small BM so I changed her and she was wide awake. It was an early breakfast for her and she ate quite well but very soon was sleeping in her chair. Back into bed for less than an hour and then up again for no apparent reason. Within a half hour she was sleeping in her chair so it was back to bed. This time she slept for close to four hour and then was wide awake again. She ate a good lunch and in a very short time was sleeping in her chair so it was back to bed. She just seemed upset or maybe she had some pain but I had no idea. The entire day was spent with short naps and then longer than normal periods of being wide awake. I suspected that maybe she has a urinary tract infection but of course problems like this always seem to occur on weekends. In desperation the hospice on-call nurse was contacted. She came, took vital signs and then suggested that maybe she should be given either morphine or Xanax (the medication which caused the 37 hour sleep). I finally agreed to give her ½ Xanax tablet but after over a half hour there was no visible effect. She was put into bed for the night over 2 hours past her normal bed time but just wouldn't sleep. Finally she was given the other half of the Xanax tablet. Within a half hour she was sleeping soundly.

We always consider that a day is 24 hours but that is not necessarily the case with my Sweetheart. Today started when she was laid in bed to sleep last evening and it will end when she is put into bed this evening. Some days may have as high as 27 hours if she went to bed early last evening and stayed up a little later than normal this evening. Yesterday when she had the problems it was a 27 hour day for her but her awake time was close to 7 hours which is extremely abnormal for her. She is normally awake just less than 3 hours each day. Her temperature was nearly normal today so I don't suspect a urinary tract infection.

Her sleep time was about normal today but it was a struggle getting her to eat and drink. I woke her a little before 11 AM and could only get her to drink about one half glass of juice. Her breakfast was a pancake but she ate less than half. Finally, she was fed some of her favorite cookies but soon was sleeping in her wheel chair. I woke her from a sound sleep at 4:30 PM and was successful in getting her to drink a reasonable amount of juice. She would only eat a small amount of her Meals on Wheels lunch. I finally resorted to an ice cream bar and more of her favorite cookies. Normally she eats well but then there are days when she just refuses. I always look forward to tomorrow and hope she will return to her normal eating and drinking habits.

On Tuesday of this week I suspected that my Sweetheart may have a Urinary Tract Infection. I was successful in getting a urine sample and called the hospice to pick it up and have it checked. I didn't hear any report and on Friday morning when the nurse came she said that yes, my Sweetheart does have a urinary tract infection. She said there was some kind of mix up on getting the report but finally late Thursday she forwarded the information to the doctor to get a prescription. It is now noon on Friday and no medication. We should have been treating the infection at least two days ago. In the future I plan to call several times each day so if there is some kind of mix up it won't prolong the process of getting medication in a timely manner.

I woke her today just before 11 AM after over 17 hours of sleep. She ate the applesauce with the medications with no problems. She drank a large glass of juice but when it came to the main meal, she just didn't want to eat. The meal was sweet and sour pork, vegetables and spiced apples. She took a few bites of each and then just refused to eat. I offered her a frosted animal cookie and she ate it with no problems. I would feed her several of the cookies but then try a bite of the main meal and she just wouldn't take a bite. She knows what she likes, what she doesn't like and just won't eat what she doesn't like. Good for her!

Last night she went to bed for the night at 5:30. She was asleep when her head hit the pillow and slept soundly until a little after 11 PM. She was fussing and just didn't seem to want to sleep. I checked and she had a bowel movement and needed changing. After she was changed, sleep would not come. She just kept tossing, turning and muttering. At about 2 AM there was another bowel movement and again she was changed but wouldn't sleep. Finally in desperation she was given half of a Xanax tablet but it didn't seem to help. She seemed like she was in pain. About 3 AM she was given some morphine which seemed to help. This morning she did eat the applesauce with the medication, wouldn't drink hardly a swallow and just refused to eat any additional food. She was put into bed and napped for 5 hours. After the nap, she ate the applesauce with the night medication, drank 2 glasses of juice, ate a limited amount of regular food but ate cookies and part of an ice cream bar. I put her back into bed for the night and she seemed to be asleep immediately.

Today was my Sweetheart's shower day. Since she frequently doesn't assist by planting her good leg when moved, two CNA's come to give her the shower. They indicated that she has a yeast infection and needs to be treated. They said that the necessary medication would be delivered before the end of the day. When I arrived home from my day off a little before 4 PM, the medication had not been delivered. The hospice was called to get a status of when it would be delivered. I was told that someone would call me back with the information. No one had called an hour later so I called again as the hospice office closes at 5 PM. A few minutes later they called and said they hoped the medication would be delivered but weren't sure. This appears to be a repeat of the urinary tract infection medication. It doesn't seem there is any sense of urgency to get medication which results in needless suffering by the patient.

The medication to treat the yeast infection was delivered about 7 PM. Naturally it was too late to do anything that evening because my Sweetheart was sound asleep for the night. The instructions on the powdered medication was to apply 3 times daily. The yeast infection is in the groin area and I just didn't know where to begin. The lady who delivered the medication was questioned and she said to wash the groin area, dry the area completely and then apply the powder. The next morning I woke my Sweetheart a half hour before I'd be leaving for my 7 hours off. It was definitely a struggle to get the powder properly applied. My helper had applied the medication later in the day so there was no need for another application that day. The next morning being shower day, I decided to let them do the application after the shower and I'd watch to see what I could learn. I did learn something. There were two shower people and they had just as much trouble getting the groin area cleaned, dried, and the powder applied.

For about the last 10 days, my Sweetheart just hasn't been doing well. It has been extremely difficult getting her to eat and drink. I have had the nagging feeling that the end is very close. Nothing has been mentioned to the other family members. This morning she woke a little after 8 with a bowel movement. She was cleaned then the work started to apply the yeast infection powder. It was a significant effort but when done, my Sweetheart seemed very alert and ready for food. She ate very well with very little coaxing. Her breakfast consisted of 1 ½ glasses of juice, a small dish of applesauce with her medications, one scrambled egg, two link sausages and finished with some frosted animal cookies. Soon after her breakfast she was tired and put down for her nap. It is the start of a very good day.

The yeast infection and the urinary tract infection are both cured. Now she has a terrible rash again on her back. We are treating it with the same ointment that was used before but it doesn't seem to be responding that well. I wash her back each morning and then apply the ointment. At night I just apply ointment.

My Sweetheart has lost her appetite and doesn't drink nearly as much liquid as she should. This morning she did drink 2 glasses of juice but wouldn't eat at all except for the applesauce used to give her medications. This evening, again she ate the applesauce but refused to drink. By doing a great deal of coaxing, she ate a small dish of ice cream, a small brownie, an ice cream bar and several cookies. If this continues, there is no doubt that she is transitioning. I'm certainly not ready, nor will I ever be ready for the last day to end.

The morning started like most other morning but she just didn't eat that well and would only drink ½ glass of juice. She napped for about 6 hours and then I had to wake her. It was really a struggle to get her to eat anything. I finally did get her to eat a small dish of applesauce with her medications, maybe 3 small bites of fish, one cookie and a small dish of ice cream. She just didn't want to eat. Again, she drank only another half glass of juice. Her total liquid intake for the day was only 1 glass. Normally she will drink about 3 glasses full each day. All of us have our days when we just don't feel like eating so I'm hoping that is the case and that she will eat and drink well tomorrow.

One of our sons gave his Mother a box of candy for Mother's Day. The big day isn't until tomorrow but I opened the candy for her today and told her who gave it and that it was for Mother's Day. She just couldn't bite the chocolate. It seems that her lower front teeth are no longer upright but are tilted back considerably. It almost impossible for her to bite something but she does well chewing on her back teeth. I cut each of two chocolates into 4 pieces and she was able to eat them with no problems.

One of our favorite meals was fried potatoes and fried trout. I acquired some freshly caught trout and today I fried potatoes and trout. After the first bite of each, there was no doubt in my mind that she knew just exactly what she was eating. She never hesitated and ate a large helping of each.

A person never knows what to expect. Two days after her fish and fried potatoes day, she just didn't want to eat anything. Her total awake time was only 30 minutes in the morning and 45minutes in the early evening. She did drink well but it was very difficult getting her to eat anything. I'm sure that as time goes on days like this will become the norm.

It was a three nap day for my Sweetheart. After her last nap she was wide awake, talkative and ate well. She spent over 30 minutes at her table playing with her toys. During the night she just didn't seem to want to sleep. She was constantly groaning as if in pain but the narcotic pain patch should prevent that from being an issue. I suspect maybe another urinary tract infection. I have been successful in getting a urine sample first thing in the morning. Hopefully we can get results as we are approaching a three day holiday weekend.

The urine sample tested positive so now we are treating another urinary tract infection. The medication is in large capsules to be given three times daily for seven days. The capsules are emptied into the apple sauce along with her morning and night medications. The applesauce has a very bitter taste with all of the medications added so some pancake syrup is added to counteract the bitterness.

We have a small television in the kitchen close to where she eats her meals. I usually have it turned on for no other reason than the company. The last few days I have positioned her wheel chair directly in front of the television so she can see the pictures while she is eating. It seems that she is more alert and does better eating her meals. I try to pick a sports program or something with action which seems to hold her interest. .

The hospital bed is located at the foot of the bed in the master bedroom. The ceiling light fixture is directly above the hospital bed so when the light is on and her eyes are open, she is looking directly at the light. This has been a concern for some time. I modified the bottom of a card board box and was able to attach it to the bottom of the fixture. This minor change has a significant effect on her comfort and really doesn't diminish the amount of light in the room. I should have made that change a long time ago.

I woke her at 9:30 this morning but she wouldn't drink hardly at all and would only eat half of the apple sauce with the morning medications. I finally just gave up and she was back into bed at 10 AM. At 2 PM she was awaken again and did manage to get her to drink a small amount and eat the remainder of the apple sauce with the morning medications. She ate maybe 2 bites of mashed potatoes and gravy and 2 bites of fried chicken. The eating was followed by a violent choking spell. I tried feeding her some ice cream but she just didn't want to eat. It was back into bed at 2:30 PM. Finally, at 5:30 PM she was wide awake, thirsty and hungry. She ate a very good meal and took her medications with no problems. She was really quite alert and was awake for over an hour.

A lady who we have known for years came to visit. Her husband has been diagnosed with dementia. She seemed very frustrated and was looking for information. She was acquainted with the lady who helps me two days a week and was looking at my "dementia journey" book that is filled with pictures and notes. Her husband has had several other health problems and it seemed to me from talking with her that she had more than her share of health problems. She currently cares for her husband who is close to six feet tall and weighs over 200 pounds. I know that she would like to continue caring for him but as his condition worsens, there is no way that she will physically be able to do the things that she needs to do. I am very fortunate that my health is good and that I am able to continue caring for my Sweetheart. I have so many memories that will be with me forever.

Yesterday was my day for cortisone shots in my left knee and left hip. They were just as painful as I remembered. As the day wore on, both the knee and hip became more painful. Both areas were iced during the evening. Sleep would not come and at about 1:30 AM, both areas were iced but didn't help. Finally, about 3 AM I dressed and went grocery shopping at the all night grocery store. Hopefully some sleep will come intermittently during the day today.

I frequently read newspaper or magazine articles about Alzheimer's and Dementia. Many of them graphically explain about the combative nature of the patients. I am blessed because of never having to cope with those problems. My Sweetheart has very mild behavior. I'm sure that I have many issues different from other patients but wandering and combativeness are not a problem.

I woke her this morning at 10 AM but she just didn't ever get fully awake. It was a big problem getting her to eat the apple sauce with her morning medicine but it was accomplished and she was put back into bed for a nap with only about 15 minutes of awake time. I tried to wake her at 2 PM, 3 PM and finally at 4 PM she was awake. She ate a very good meal and then an ice cream bar. She ate a few cookies and another ice cream bar. At 5 PM she was napping in her wheel chair so it was back to bed for the night. Her total awake time for the day was only 1 hour 15 minutes.

There was really no apparent signs of her having a urinary tract infection but I just suspected there was something wrong. When she first wakes in the morning is the time when I've been able to get a good urine sample. It was a Monday morning and when she started to wake-up, she had a huge bowel movement and so getting a good sample was not an option. The following morning it was no problem.

The hospice nurse was contacted and when she looked at the sample her immediate reaction was that she definitely has a UTI. After testing, her doctor was notified and a prescription delivered before the end of the day. The final laboratory results showed that a different prescription was needed and it was delivered late Friday afternoon. The instructions are to give one capsule 4 times daily. Giving her medications three times daily is no problem but with her average awake time being less than 3 hours each day, the 4 times daily is a definite challenge.

Her morning nap is normally at least 4 hours but after only one hour today she was pulling at the sheets and muttering. I wasn't sure why she was not sleeping soundly. I finally decided to check and see if she needed her diaper changed. Yes, she had a large bowel movement and was trying to tell me to change her diaper but I just wasn't listening.

Thursday was the last day for my helper. She is moving out of state and will be sorely missed as she has been helping care for my Sweetheart for over 52 months. I am now working with a home care agency and have been assigned a new person starting this next week. She came for an orientation and I'm sure she will work out well. She has significant experience in nursing and also in care giving.

She just wouldn't wake-up this morning. It was difficult getting her into the wheel chair because she wouldn't plant her left leg. As always, she was thirsty and drank most of her juice but wouldn't take even one bite of the apple sauce with her medications. I tried washing her face with a cold and wet cloth but without success. Finally, she was just put back into her hospital bed to sleep. When she wakes at mid-day, she will be given the apple sauce with the medications before she gets her regular noon day meal.

I just finished treating a urinary tract infection on a Friday. The following week it seemed that things just weren't quite the way they should be so I got another urine specimen. Now we are treating another urinary tract infection starting less than a week after completing the last.

My new caregiver helper worked on Wednesday and Thursday of this week. Things seemed to go well but she did want a slider board to assist in transferring my Sweetheart from the bed to the wheel chair.

After she left on Thursday, I walked into the dark bedroom to put something away and crashed into the wheel chair that she had left parked in the main pathway rather than the normal place. I fell and injured my right arm and ended up in the emergency room. Also, she had put my Sweetheart to bed with her dress still on which is never done. The next day the home health people called and said she had quit because it was too much lifting for her. Now, the following Tuesday, I will be training another caregiver to help.

And thus ended the eleventh day.

CHAPTER 12

ᘙᘙᘙᘙᘙᘙ

The Last Day

Less than a week ago we finished treating a urinary tract infection for my Sweetheart. Friday morning I had the feeling that we needed a urine sample because she was just acting a little strange. Sure enough, another urinary tract infection. By noon a medication was delivered. Hopefully this is the correct medication but we will not know for sure until the final laboratory results are received.

The Meals on Wheels lunch today was fried chicken strips but they just didn't have much taste for my Sweetheart. A sauce was furnished with the meal but tasted quite strong and spicy. One bite with that sauce was more than enough and she just refused to have another. I then tried using Thousand Island salad dressing but again, only one bite was enough. Finally, some Sweet and Sour sauce was tried and that was the magic bullet. She ate both strips without any further hesitation. She may not have much of a mind but she still knows what she likes and what she dislikes.

In addition to the urinary tract infection, she now has another yeast infection. I notified the hospice on-call nurse and she confirmed the yeast infection and gave me some instruction on treatment. My Sweetheart was just very miserable and in desperation she was given a Xanax (.25 mg) tablet. She was able to go to sleep and slept well. The next morning she just didn't want to wake-up. It was very difficult getting her to take the necessary medications. She drank three glasses of juice, ate two very small dishes of apple sauce, one ice cream bar and just a few cookies for her total intake for the day. It was not a wise choice giving her the Xanax tablet.

She still has another urinary tract infection in less than a week after we finished treating the last one. Also, the yeast infection just doesn't seem to be improving. The nurse checked her this morning and ordered some internal medication as well as the powder. The internal medication must be taken once each day for seven days. I feel so sorry for my Sweetheart but just don't know what to do to help her.

I usually check her temperature each time she is helped out of bed. Her temperature with an ear thermometer normally runs between 98.6 and 99.1. Tuesday evening the temperature showed 99.6 and it was time to get a urine sample. From past experience the best time to get a urine sample from my Sweetheart is when she first gets out of bed in the morning. It was one of my golf days and my helper indicated that the hospice picked up the sample and told her to inform me that 99.6 was not a fever and I shouldn't be concerned. I know my Sweetheart better than anyone and just seem to have a feeling that something is wrong. Well, later in the day a prescription was delivered to treat a urinary tract infection. One capsule three times daily is the dosage. I had her morning medications mixed with a small amount of yogurt but she just wouldn't take even one bite. The yogurt with her medications was put into her morning glass of orange juice, mixed thoroughly, and she drank every drop.

On a Sunday afternoon, two of our sons were visiting and their Mother was still napping. I woke her from the nap and called our two sons to come and observe what was required to change her diaper, move her to the wheel chair and finish dressing her. One of our sons indicated he didn't need to observe because he already knew but came to the bedroom anyway. Five days later she had just eaten the evening meal when I became very ill. I called the youngest son and told him he needed to come and care for his Mother because I needed to go to the hospital emergency room. A short time later, I called him from the hospital and informed him that I was being admitted and that he was now the caregiver until further notice. Late the following day another son, not living in the area, arrived with his wife and two grown daughters to assist in the care giving. I was hospitalized for four days and they did well caring for my Sweetheart. This is just another example of the importance of a backup plan.

The Meals on Wheels meal today was meat loaf, mac & cheese, and peas. As I gave her each bite it was identified as the food was brought to her mouth. When I attempted to give her the second bite of peas, she refused to open her mouth but continued to eat the meat loaf and mac & cheese. Finally, she had apparently had her fill and would no longer open her mouth. Then I asked if she would like a cookie and she immediately opened her mouth. She continued to eat cookies until she had her fill. Sometimes we think that people with Alzheimer's really don't understand very much but I'm sure they understand more than we think they understand.

In the evening day before yesterday she was very nervous and sleep would not come. After my earlier experience with Xanax .25 mg, I didn't want to give her another. I took one of the .25 mg tablets and cut it in half, put it in a small amount of freezer jam and she swallowed it without any problems. A little later she was sound asleep. The next morning she would not wake up. She wouldn't wake for the shower or the evening meal. Her total food and drink consumption was minimal. About 8 PM that evening she needed changed because of a large bowel movement and in the process she was wide awake. She was put into the wheel chair and taken to the kitchen where she ate a large helping of ice cream and a large brownie. She also drank nearly two glasses of cranberry juice. On those very restless days Xanax in even a very small dosage does not appear to be a good option.

My regular caregiver needed a few days off so a substitute was sent. She was given some training a few days before. On her first morning, a Saturday, she was scheduled to arrive at 7:30 AM. When she didn't arrive the on-call scheduler was contacted. She called me back in just a few minutes and indicated the caregiver would arrive in about 15 minutes. We are currently treating my Sweetheart for another urinary tract infection and is given one capsule 3 times daily. I told the caregiver that she needed to give her the mid-day capsule. When I questioned her after I had returned, she indicated that the mid-day capsule had not been given. I gave her the medication with the evening meal and later that evening she woke and was given another capsule. The next morning when the caregiver came, she told me that she had given her the mid-day capsule the day before.

The medication being given for the UTI was because of a preliminary test which showed an infection. The specimen had been submitted to the lab on Friday morning. When the nurse came on Monday she indicated that the lab report had not been received. Tuesday morning the nurse was contacted and indicated that the lab report had been received and that a different medication was needed. The new medication will be delivered today and will require one tablet 2 times daily for 10 days. My Sweetheart has a UTI and has been taking the wrong medication for 4 days. Not good.

She finally finished the last of the UTI medicine and hopefully we won't have a repeat for a little while. She has been very alert and eaten very well for the last several days. The average sleep time hasn't changed much and for last month it was 21.1 hours average each day. She has completed 4 years and 7 months as a hospice patient and she just doesn't seem to be changing much. I am so fortunate that she has a good disposition and don't have to contend with combative issues.

Now she has developed a large cyst on her lower back. It was discovered on a Monday at the time the hospice nurse was visiting. She didn't seem concerned about the cyst and didn't suggest any treatment. A little later in the day I visited a local pharmacy and purchased a drawing ointment. It was applied twice daily for 5 days and didn't seem to have any effect. A different nurse visited on Friday and she was questioned about a possible treatment. I suggested that she take a picture and ask the hospice doctor what treatment would be appropriate. She later informed me that the doctor indicated that no treatment was necessary. I looked on the internet for a suggested treatment and it indicated that wet heat for 20-30 minutes several times each day. It appears to be having a positive effect.

I talked with the hospice about a flu shot for my Sweetheart. The pharmacy they use informed me that I would need to pay $34.99 for the shot because they were unable to bill Medicare where my Sweetheart is a hospice patient. I contacted Medicare and asked if the flu shot would be covered under Medicare Part B where she was a hospice patient. They indicated that it would be covered. Apparently I can take my Sweetheart to a grocery store or pharmacy where they give flu shots and the total cost will be covered by Medicare but hospice cannot get the serum and administer the shot. Where she is bedridden, it is just too difficult to try and transport her to a place where the shot can be given. I'll submit a claim to Medicare and attempt to get reimbursed for the cost of the flu shot. I will be surprised if they reimburse anything.

When I went in to wake my Sweetheart this morning, the whole side of her face was covered with blood. She had bitten her lip and was bleeding profusely. It is not uncommon for her to bite her lip but she has never bitten it so it bled so freely.

The helper that I have now for two days each week called me one day and suggested that I start giving my Sweetheart some cranberry juice. She indicated that I should get the 100% juice rather than the watered down version. A few days later I bought the juice and have been giving her at least a full glass each day. We've had no urinary tract infections to contend with since starting the cranberry juice. Could it be that the cranberry juice is responsible for her being UTI free?

Daylight savings time just ended again. I don't know how to reset my own internal clock and it takes me at least a month to adjust to the time change. My Sweetheart is still operating on the old time schedule and I'm sure it will take her a considerable time to adjust. I wish that one time would be selected and then leave it alone. It is very disrupting to change twice yearly.

We had a houseful of people at Thanksgiving with our family of children, grandchildren, great grandchildren and spouses all in attendance. Seldom are we able to have everyone at the same place at the same time. I was amazed at how well my Sweetheart tolerated everything. Just before the big dinner it was picture taking time. I'd gotten her up from her nap a short time before and she was wide awake. She stayed wide awake through dinner and ate very well. After the dinner she stayed awake almost another hour and then it was nap time.

She has been so alert and eaten so well for several weeks now that it is unbelievable.

The day following Thanksgiving was her normal shower day. Normally the hospice sends two CNA's to give the showers but this time, only one was available. I needed to do the lifting to get her onto the shower chair and also back into the wheel chair. During the process, she must have bumped her big toe on one foot and it was bleeding around the toe nail. Several years ago that toe nail needed removed and when it grew back it was extremely thick. As it was examined closer, it was almost ready to fall off. The toe nail was removed and bandaged. It didn't seem that she had any pain or discomfort during the whole process.

For several days she has been extremely alert and eaten very well. Today that was not the case. I tried to wake her at 9 AM and did manage to get her to drink a half glass of juice and take her morning medications. I tried to feed her some lunch about 12:30 today but only one bite and a few swallows of juice, then back into bed. Finally at 3 PM she seemed to be stirring and she did eat and drink quite well. It was back into bed at 4 PM where she slept 17 hours. When she woke, she was hungry and thirsty. Again at 1 PM she was awake and ate a very large lunch. We just take things a few hours at a time because there is no way to predict.

The regular nurse comes each Monday and Friday morning and normally arrives by about 8:15. This particular morning, no nurse. The hospice called a short time later and informed me that the regular nurse was ill and another would be visiting. He had made a visit about a year earlier and he remarked that he could see a significant difference since his last visit.

She seldom speaks and when she does it is usually only one word. This morning when she would try to speak she just couldn't make a sound. She has just a terrible cold and is extremely congested. Her temperature has also been elevated. I have been giving her over-the-counter daytime cold medication four times daily. That medication has Tylenol but not of sufficient strength so an additional 500 mg tablet has been added to each dosage. After four days she seems to be improving and has regained her appetite. Hopefully she continues to improve.

Today is Christmas Day and we ordered some her favorite Chinese food. This morning she was awakened at 9:15 and ate well but it was with significant effort. She did drink 2 ½ glasses of juice. When lunch time arrived she was awakened at 1:30 PM and just didn't seem hungry at all. She drank another glass of juice but would hardly eat a bite. Finally, she was just put back into bed for her nap. I am concerned that she may be transitioning but of course I've had those concerned in the past.

The lady that helped me two days each week from March 2013 until July 2017 moved out of state. She and her family returned to this area for a visit during the holidays. Yesterday she came to visit and my Sweetheart was sleeping. A short time later she was awake and needed her diaper changed. When she was moved to a sitting position on the side of the bed, the lady moved directly in front of her and started talking. My Sweetheart gave her a look of recognition and a smile. She seldom smiles for anyone. For at least a moment, she definitely knew who had come to visit.

New Years day came to a close and she routinely went to bed at the regular hour. At 2:30 AM the following morning she began coughing and choking. I gave her a drink with some cold medication in it and she seemed to be doing well. At 5:30 AM she had a severe coughing spell and her temperature was 100.4. More cold medication and 500 mg Tylenol were given and the temperature seemed to drop. She slept until 10 AM ate a small breakfast with more cold medication and drank two glasses of juice. When I went to wake her at 2 PM for her lunch, she sounded terrible and seemed to be choking. Her temperature was 101.4. As I was transferring her from the bed to the wheel chair, she slipped and slid to the floor. The hospice was notified and help was sent to get her off the floor and into the wheel chair. It was an easy fall with no injuries. She ate a very small mid-day meal, drank 1 ½ glasses of juice with more cold medication and Tylenol The nurse believes that she is transitioning. It doesn't look good to me for her to change so drastically in less than 24 hours.

She was put into bed for the night a little before 6 and the head of the hospital bed was raised. She seemed to be resting well. A short time later I noticed that she was very congested and gasping for breath. The hospital bed was raised more but didn't seem to help. She was taken out of the hospital bed and put into the wheel chair with her dress on. A large towel was wrapped around her legs and a shawl placed over her upper body. I put a slider board behind her to keep her head from falling back. A large vaporizer was sat on the floor beside her and hopefully will give her some relief. It may be necessary to leave her in the wheel chair for the entire night. I'm thinking it may be a short night for us both.

I checked her periodically in the wheel chair and she seemed to be doing well. About 9 PM when she was checked it was noted that she had a large runny bowel movement that ran down both legs and onto the floor. She was moved to the bed and cleaned. She was washed thoroughly and given clean underclothes.

She had a terrible cough and seemed to have severe chest congestion. A little later the on-call hospice nurse was contacted and she made a visit. She indicated that my Sweetheart was transitioning and that she needed Morphine every two hours to help her breathe easier and prevent undue suffering. She finished her visit at 12:30 AM and then came back at 6 AM the next morning to follow-up. My Sweetheart won't drink or eat anything. Her temperature is elevated and we have finally gotten some Tylenol suppositories as well as some medication to help the congestion. I've tried repeatedly to give her something to drink without success. During the last two days she has been visited at least two times by the on-call nurse and also by her regular hospice nurse. The regular hospice nurse was asked today how long transitions normally last? Her response was that in her patients it normally would take about two weeks but she didn't think it would take nearly that long with my Sweetheart. I have tried to keep our three sons informed by email and telephone.

The hospice nurse indicated that in many instances that patients in transition seem to linger because they are awaiting goodbyes and confirmation that it is OK to leave the living. She strongly suggested that family members be contacted and that they have an opportunity to come and spend some time with my Sweetheart. She went on to say that if family members could not personally come to visit that a telephone call on a speaker telephone held close to her ear would be a good alternative. She went on to say that hearing was the last of the senses to leave a patient. That same day a granddaughter in a far away state called and talked to her grandmother on the speaker phone. Then a little later in the day, one of our sons who lives about 400 miles away, called and talked to his Mom on the speaker phone and told her goodbye.

The morning following my son's goodbye to his Mom over the telephone, he sent an email that he and the family were en route to visit. A little later in the day they arrived, our oldest son and his wife, our youngest son, my Sweetheart's brother his wife and their two grown daughters all visited and said their goodbyes. My Sweetheart is still with us two days later. She is given medication normally every two hours but at times hourly to prevent undue suffering. It is a difficult time for all but I will never be ready for her passing.

My Sweetheart took only 2 small pills in the morning and 2 different pills at night plus a narcotic pain patch that was changed every 3 days. Of those medications, the pain patch is the only one being used. The transition medications are all liquid with one to help dissipate the congestion, one for agitation, and morphine for pain. In addition, we have a Tylenol suppository for fever control. The medication given for congestion is in a very small bottle similar to an eye drop bottle and the normal dosage is 2 drops. The container is made of a material making it impossible to determine the amount remaining. It was mid-afternoon and time for medication. As I attempted to put two drops in a spoon, nothing but air bubbles. No problem, I knew that a new prescription was at a local pharmacy awaiting pickup. It was a Saturday afternoon and I went to the pharmacy but was shocked when it had closed for the weekend at 2 PM. The on-call nurse was contacted and told of the problem. A short time later she was at our door with the necessary medications.

Tonight she was given a Tylenol suppository for fever control. During the process of inserting the suppository, it was noted that she has two sores on one knee, one of which it down to the muscle. We have been putting a small folded blanket between her knees to prevent that but it hasn't worked. Also, it was noted that she has several places in the area of her tailbone where the skin is breaking down into a sore. The hospice nurse had bandages that were placed over the areas and hopefully will provide some protection. Each time that we roll her onto her right side, she has discharged a green looking bile solution from her mouth. Things are just not good and it is becoming more and more difficult for me each day. Hopefully the good Lord above will take her so she will no longer have to endure the suffering. It is just so sad to witness it and be helpless to do anything about her suffering.

The bandages were changed today and it was extremely difficult for her being rolled from side to side. Again, there was the discharge of the green colored solution. She was choking and gasping during the entire time. Finally she was laid straight in the bed, covered with a sheet and the head of the bed elevated. In just a short time she was resting and looked very comfortable.

The on call nurse arrived about 6 PM and stayed until almost 9 PM. She indicated that she was sure that my Sweetheart would leave us sometime during the night. She told me to check on her frequently and continue giving medications. She said that when she passed on that I needed to note the time and then call the regular office number and the afterhours answering service would contact her. There are times when no life is detected but then she would take a deep breath. At 6 AM the following morning the nurse called to check on my Sweetheart's status. About 7 AM she visited and stayed until the regular nurse arrived. About 10 AM the CNA's came to give the bed bath. There was some wound dressings that needed changing. It was a very difficult process for my Sweetheart with her laying on her side, gasping for breath and frequently having the green looking discharge come from her mouth. The past 10 days have been an extremely difficult time for me and I'm sure it won't get any easier until she passes.

I was checking her frequently and she was just gasping for breath and had that terrible gurgling sound in her throat. I felt so helpless because there was just nothing that I could do to help. A little after 1:30 PM, a knock came at the door and it was my Sweetheart's brother. We went into her room and stood by her for a short time and then went to the living room to visit. Less than 5 minutes later I returned to her room and she had passed away. I felt so sad but also relieved because she was no longer fighting for breath. The hospice nurse was call and when she arrived I told her that it was 1:50 PM when she stopped breathing. The nurse called the funeral home and a short time later they arrived and removed the body. All the necessary information was completed which was required for issuance of the death certificate. The final transition started on January 2nd and my Sweetheart passed away on January 10th. Here are the final weight and sleep graphs for the time that they were maintained:

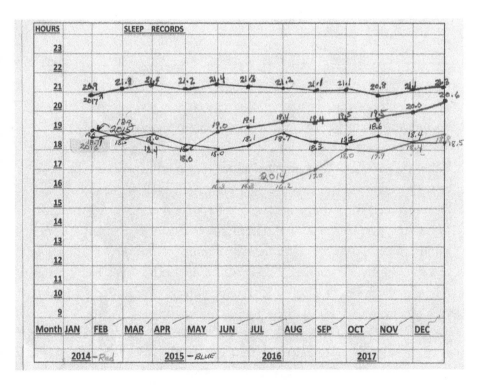

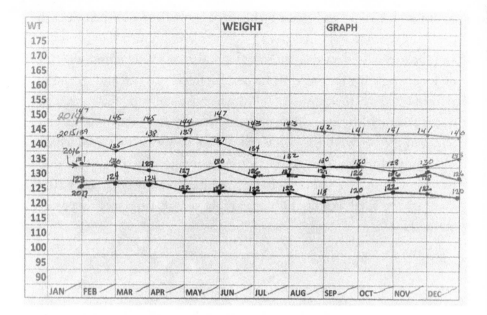

It is interesting to note that each year the weight continued to decline and each year the average sleep time per day increased.

For the past two days my efforts have been directed to funeral and burial preparation. We had purchased a pre-paid funeral several years ago. Our cemetery plots were also purchased and the headstone has been installed with all the necessary information except dates of death. My Sweetheart was able to choose her own casket at a time when her mind was still sharp. There were two musical numbers during her funeral. Both were done extremely well. One of the songs had a poem that was narrated with soft background music. To me the poem was very touching and the last part goes as follows:

Should You Go First
by Albert Kennedy Rowswell

Should you go first and I remain,
one thing I'll have you do:
Walk slowly down that long long path,
for soon I'll follow you.

I want to know each step you take,
so I may take the same.
For someday down that lonely road
you'll hear me call your name.

When I leave the bedroom in the mornings, soft music is automatically started the way it has been done for over 4 years. I frequently find myself rising from my chair to go check on my Sweetheart.

Wonders never cease! I don't have the death certificates yet but decided to call the insurance company to notify them of my Sweetheart's death. I wanted to get the necessary information so the claim could be submitted properly. I was on hold a very long time but when my call was finally answered I gave her name, policy number and date of death. I again was placed on hold but only for a very short time. The lady then informed me that she was able to find the death notice on line and that no death certificate would be needed. She went on to say that the full proceeds would be mailed by regular mail today.

We had a public viewing late afternoon on Sunday with the funeral being held the following day. Everything was just perfect for the funeral. Here it is, the middle of January and normally we would have extreme cold and the ground would be snow covered. At the time of burial, the temperature was close to 40 degrees and we had no snow at all. How fortunate can a person be.

I didn't realize that our house was so empty and quiet as it is today. My Sweetheart seldom made any sound at all but her presence just gave a feeling of warmth. Her table in front of the TV is still intact with the wheel chair sitting at the table. I'll just leave things in place until I feel it is time to remove them.

I went to the Social Security office today to claim the death benefit. The funeral home had said that all the death information was on line and no death certificate was needed. The first thing that I was asked was for a death certificate. I asked if they couldn't verify the information on line. They said no but wanted a copy of our marriage license. A person should call me at 11 AM in two days to finish the process over the telephone. The next thing was to contact Veterans Administration and inform them of the death so my disability pension could be reduced. They asked several questions but refused to even try for an on line verification of the death. It seems very strange that so much information is needed to reduce the payment to me. I guess I just don't understand.

I know of several things that need to be done after her death and am sure that there will be several more. A copy of the death certificate is needed by each bank and credit union where we have accounts. I need to check my life insurance policies and in some cases change the beneficiary. I receive two different retirements and provided survivor benefits on both. That needs to be changed as there is no one living that qualifies for survivor benefits.

My Sweetheart passed away on January 10, 2018. Christmas of 2018 was my first Christmas without my Sweetheart. Two days before Christmas I found this poem and it was very appropriate.

MY FIRST CHRISTMAS IN HEAVEN
Author Unknown

I see the many Christmas trees around the world below,
With tiny lights like heavens stars reflecting on the snow.
The sight is so spectacular pleas wipe away that tear,
For I'll be spending Christmas with Jesus Christ this year.

I hear the many Christmas songs that people hold so dear,
But the sound of music can't compare with
the Christmas choir up here.
I have no words to tell you the joy their voices bring,
For it's beyond description to hear the angels sing.

I know how much you miss me. I see the pain inside your heart.
But I am not so far away. We really aren't apart.
So be happy for me dear ones. You know I hold you dear.
And be glad I'm spending Christmas with Jesus Christ this year.

I send you each a special gift from my heavenly home above.
I send you each a memory of my undying love.
After all "LOVE" is a gift more precious than pure gold.
It was always most important in the stories Jesus told.

Please love and keep each other as my Father said to do,
For I can't count the blessings or the love he has for each of you.
So have a Merry Christmas and wipe away that tear,
Remember, I'm spending Christmas with Jesus Christ this year.

Caring for my Sweetheart really began over 9 years ago with the last 4 years and 10 months being a hospice patient. It was a long road but given the opportunity to do it again, I wouldn't hesitate even for a minute. It was the right thing to do and I was blessed with good health for the entire time. She was able to remain in her own home and be cared for by loved ones. I am convinced that was a great contributing factor for her longevity. I know that there is a life hereafter and someday we will be together again. I will be looking forward to that day with great anticipation.

And thus ended the last day.